"True to the central understandings of cr
Freire, Darder, Steinberg, and Giroux, amo
engaging essays, moves from a critical analy
problematiques to meaningful possibilities ... ...w
generation of critical pedagogues represented here, focus on pain, suffering
and trauma, and yet, skilfully and subversively construct a pedagogy based
on a counter-narrative – one that is so much needed in present neoliberal,
fatalist, and pandemic times. The emotive, rational, and poetic are very positively intertwined to offer a strong and courageous voice to a renewed form
of critical pedagogy."

– **John P. Portelli, PhD**, Professor Emeritus,
Ontario Institute for Studies in Education,
University of Toronto

"Weaved throughout *Counternarratives of Pain and Suffering as Critical
Pedagogy* are powerful stories of triumph that disrupt discursive practices
in educational contexts. The book amplifies the voices of Black, Indigenous,
and People of Colour (BIPOC) and offers analyses of lived experiences negotiating identities, resisting oppression, and confronting stereotypes. Readers
are invited to break through the cycle of silence and consider who benefits
when dominant ideologies are not challenged. Connected to current social
landscapes, the book offers a pedagogical framework of hope, possibilities,
and resiliency to achieve transformational change and affirms the need for
diversity, equity, and inclusion in academic spaces."

– **Gaëtane Jean-Marie, PhD**, Dean and
Professor of Educational Leadership, College
of Education, Rowan University

"Eizadirad, Campbell, and Sider offer a timely and necessary salve to historical and ongoing wounds of pain, trauma, and suffering. Their book reveals
confessions as truth-telling that narrate emotional, physical, and spiritual
injuries inflicted by oppression as well as individual and collective acts of
resistance, resilience, care, and compassion. Each chapter unfolds counternarratives that are difficult to read, yet we need to bear their lessons to not
only survive but also thrive. For our well-being and critical solidarity, this
book is a compelling read in these challenging times!"

– **Roland Sintos Coloma, PhD**, Professor,
Division of Teacher Education,
Wayne State University

"This volume provides a rare opportunity to reflect on one's narrative of
pain and suffering from a theoretical standpoint. As the editor's state: 'We
encourage you to reflect on your own life and experiences to begin constructively engaging with your own pain, suffering, and trauma.' Each chapter is
unique and has a specific message for the reader. No one reading this book
can escape the importance of interrogating the institutional, structural, and
societal visible and invisible ways that inflict pain and suffering. The chapters interweave complex and systemic ways that pain finds spaces and bodies

to manifest itself and re-appear in different forms in the life of individuals. This is the first time I have a read a book that articulates engaging with pain, suffering, and trauma so well and constructively. This unique book is a must read for all of us!"

– **Njoki Wane, PhD**, Professor and Chair of
Social Justice Education Department, Ontario
Institute for Studies in Education,
University of Toronto

Counternarratives of Pain and Suffering as Critical Pedagogy

Foregrounding diverse lived experiences and non-dominant forms of knowledge, this edited volume showcases ways in which narrating and sharing stories of pain and suffering can be engaged as critical pedagogy to challenge oppression and inequity in educational contexts.

The volume illustrates the need to consider both the act of narrating and the experience of bearing witness to narration to harness the full transformative potentials of counternarratives in disrupting oppressive practices. Chapters are divided into three parts – "Telling and Reliving Trauma as Pedagogy," "Pedagogies of Overcoming Silence," and "Forgetting as Pedagogy" – illustrating a range of relational pedagogical and methodological approaches, including journaling, poetry, and arts-based narrative inquiry.

The authors make the argument that the language of pain and suffering is universal, hence its potential as critical pedagogy for transformative and therapeutic teaching and learning. Readers are encouraged to reflect on their own lived experiences to constructively engage with their pain, suffering, and trauma. Focusing on trauma-informed non-hegemonic storytelling and transformative pedagogies, this volume will be of interest to students, faculty, scholars, and community members with an interest in advancing anti-oppressive and social justice education.

Ardavan Eizadirad is Assistant Professor in the Faculty of Education at Wilfrid Laurier University and an instructor at the Ontario Institute for Studies in Education at the University of Toronto, Canada. He is also the founder and director of *EDIcation Consulting* (www.edication.org) offering equity, diversity, and inclusion training to organizations.

Andrew B. Campbell is Adjunct Assistant Professor at Queen's University in the Professional Master of Education Program and a faculty member at the Ontario Institute for Studies in Education at the University of Toronto, Canada. He has taught at all levels of the education system for the last 25 years in Jamaica, Bahamas, and Canada, and is also known as Dr. ABC (https://drabc.ca/).

Steve Sider is a Professor in the Faculty of Education at Wilfrid Laurier University, Canada. He is the past president of the Comparative and International Education Society of Canada and the current director of the Centre for Leading Research in Education at Wilfrid Laurier.

Routledge Research in Educational Equality and Diversity

Books in the series include:

The Hidden Academic Curriculum and Inequality in Early Education
How Class, Race, Teacher Interactions, and Friendship Influence Student Success
Karen Phelan Kozlowski

Applying Anzalduan Frameworks to Understand Transnational Youth Identities
Bridging Culture, Language, and Schooling at the US-Mexican Border
Edited by G. Sue Kasun and Irasema Mora-Pablo

Advancing Educational Equity for Students of Mexican Descent
Creating an Asset-based Bicultural Continuum Model
Edited by Andrea Romero and Iliana Reyes

The Lived Experiences of Filipinx American Teachers in the U.S.
A Hermeneutic Phenomenological Study
Eleonor G. Castillo

Multiculturalism, Educational Inclusion, and Connectedness
Wellbeing, Ethnicity, and Identity among Chinese, South, and Southeast Asian Students
Celeste Yuen

Counternarratives of Pain and Suffering as Critical Pedagogy
Disrupting Oppression in Educational Contexts
Edited by Ardavan Eizadirad, Andrew B. Campbell, and Steve Sider

Global Perspectives on Microaggressions in Higher Education
Understanding and Combating Covert Violence in Universities
Edited by Christine L. Cho and Julie K. Corkett

For more information about this series, please visit: www.routledge.com/Routledge-Research-in-Educational-Equality-and-Diversity/book-series/RREED

Counternarratives of Pain and Suffering as Critical Pedagogy

Disrupting Oppression in Educational Contexts

Ardavan Eizadirad, Andrew B. Campbell, and Steve Sider

Routledge
Taylor & Francis Group

NEW YORK AND LONDON

First published 2023
by Routledge
605 Third Avenue, New York, NY 10158

and by Routledge
4 Park Square, Milton Park, Abingdon, Oxon, OX14 4RN

Routledge is an imprint of the Taylor & Francis Group, an informa business

© 2023 selection and editorial matter, Ardavan Eizadirad, Andrew B. Campbell, and Steve Sider; individual chapters, the contributors

The right of Ardavan Eizadirad, Andrew B. Campbell, and Steve Sider to be identified as the authors of the editorial material, and of the authors for their individual chapters, has been asserted in accordance with sections 77 and 78 of the Copyright, Designs and Patents Act 1988.

Library of Congress Cataloging-in-Publication Data
A catalog record for this title has been requested

ISBN: 9781032070858 (hbk)
ISBN: 9781032070889 (pbk)
ISBN: 9781003205296 (ebk)

DOI: 10.4324/9781003205296

Typeset in Sabon
by Deanta Global Publishing Services, Chennai, India

I dedicate this book to my ancestors, family, friends, colleagues, life-partner Ciara, and haters who have driven me to constantly grow and explore my relations to the land and people from all walks of life. Particularly, I am grateful to everyone who has helped me embrace my emotions and spirituality to cope with trauma and negative events more constructively. Those caring relationships facilitated healing to become an intentional disruptor as a form of activism to stand up to injustice. I further dedicate this book to all the families torn by war, parents who had to bury their children, and all the hoods around the world who feel neglected and silenced as a community. Institutions, including schools, need to do better and listen to the stories of pain and suffering shared by identities from equity-deserving groups. Let us indulge in our emotions, trauma, wounds, and scars, and harness energy from the pain and passion to mobilize for systemic change and make new friends along the way.

Ardavan Eizadirad

Throughout writing this book one thing that resonated with me is the idea of relationships – not just how we begin them, but how we nurture and sustain them. In a world where we can easily get distracted by "stuff," I am happy to know I have caring relationships. I wish to stop and acknowledge those people who have been in authentic relationships with me, especially in the last three years where I navigated challenging relationships more than ever to ensure my personal well-being, professional growth, and community connections. I started to list names and had to delete them. I would have needed more lines than this book would afford me. In that moment, at 7:13 am on September 30, 2021, I stopped, breathed, wiped away a tear, and smiled knowing in all the things I have, I do have caring relationships. For those who have been in relationships with me, you know yourself, you know your name would have been listed here, and you have heard my voice saying thanks multiple times. Again, I say thanks!

Andrew B. Campbell

I am learning. I want to acknowledge those who have helped me learn through my life journey: my grandfather, grade 6 teacher, and a grade 10 student who taught me an important lesson about privilege and perspective, amongst many others. I am continuing to learn and I want to thank Ardavan and Andrew, the co-editors of this book, for serving as guides in this learning process.

Steve Sider

Contents

Foreword xi
Contributors xiii

1 Centring Pedagogies of Pain and Suffering by Embracing Our
  Wounds and Scars 1
  ARDAVAN EIZADIRAD, ANDREW B. CAMPBELL, AND STEVE SIDER

PART 1
Telling and Reliving Trauma as Pedagogy 15

2 Cultivating Brave Spaces to Take Risks to Challenge Systemic
  Oppression 19
  ANDREW B. CAMPBELL AND ARDAVAN EIZADIRAD

3 Moving from Oppression to Opportunity: Bringing Light to
  Educational and Historical Contexts in Critical Pedagogy 38
  ALLYSON L. WATSON, AMEENAH SHAKIR, SUNDRA D. KINCEY,
  REGINALD K. ELLIS, AND DARIUS J. YOUNG

4 Storying Vulnerability: Creating Conditions for Generative
  Relationality in International Experiential Service Learning 52
  JESSICA VORSTERMANS

PART 2
Pedagogies of Overcoming Silence 67

5 Co-Composing Poetic and Arts-Based Narratives:
  Un-Silencing and Honouring Our Voices as Women Academics 71
  ANITA LAFFERTY AND JULIE A. MOONEY

 6 Self-Location as a Disruptive Counternarrative in Teaching
   and Learning   91
   KATERI MARIE MARANDOLA

 7 Engaging in Ethical Discourse: An Autoethnography of a
   Black Student's Journey to Self-Identity   105
   ALICIA NOREIGA

 8 Passing the Grade: Experiences of Black Males in Secondary
   Schools in Ontario, Canada   122
   DANIEL LUMSDEN

PART 3
Forgetting as Pedagogy   139

 9 Sacred Tears: Indigenous Women's Healing Journey of
   Mobilization for Educational Systemic Change   143
   SHARLA MSKOKII PELTIER AND CHARIS AUGER

10 Remembering Other Ways to Live: The Healing Energy that
   Flows from Sacred Ecology   163
   ZAHRA KASAMALI

11 Easing Anxiety for Adults in Higher Education: Regaining Self
   within Subversive, Interdisciplinary Bibliotherapy, and Visual
   Journaling   182
   CHRISTINA BELCHER

12 Poetic Justice: Healing and Disrupting Systemic Oppression in
   Education through Critical Pedagogy   199
   ARDAVAN EIZADIRAD

   Index   205

Foreword

The discourse based on discrimination, marginalization, and oppression has always been difficult to engage in due to the pain, trauma, and suffering it engenders. This may be due to the history of the untold harm meted out to racialized folks, particularly Black, Indigenous, and People of Colour, over a period of centuries. Canada and the United States, as well as other countries, have an unrecorded history of untold atrocities, which over the years have negatively impacted these nations. Despite changes in Jim Crow and racist laws, we continue to observe a system that covertly, and often overtly, reeks of racism in every shape and form within institutions and in our communities.

As a racialized scholar, social worker, and commentator who has published, taught, and commented on issues relating to domination, racism, intolerance, and inequity, particularly with regard to the mental health system, I find this book enriching, refreshing, and timely. I believe this book will not only model and highlight the work of social justice-oriented faculty in the academy but also encourage students of colour to overcome several roadblocks that often stifle their success. In several ways, this book is also laying the foundation for the impact of equity, diversity, and inclusivity work in Canada, the United States, and other parts of the world.

This book, edited by Ardavan Eizadirad, Andrew B. Campbell, and Steve Sider, explores the pain, trauma, and suffering experienced by marginalized communities in educational systems in the Western world. The authors pose difficult questions and recommend that in the spirit of openness and accountability and vulnerability, we find ways to deal with the difficult past. The book asks whether there are any spaces for racialized folks in an environment where they are only seen but not heard. The authors endorse embracing intentional influences of Black and other minoritized histories and pedagogies. This would include Black and Afrocentric ways of knowing to counter the current Eurocentric pedagogy, which often paves way for the Global North and South dichotomy. In this social construct, the Global North is seen as the helper or the "white saviour" bringing deliverance to the Global South.

The authors highlight challenges faced by racialized folks who are often silenced in the academic space. There is a sense of patriarchy in the academic sphere where preference is often given to dominant members who are empowered to steer the oars of academic discourse in their predominantly Eurocentric direction. How then do we steer the compass of educational engagement in the right direction? Has the time come for educators to embrace the principle of self-location? We need dialogue to disrupt the Eurocentric educational system, which tends to marginalize and oppress racialized individuals, particularly voices of Black, Indigenous, and People of Colour. The systemic racism permeating our educational system makes it difficult for racialized identities to belong. Thus, would developing the human spirit through the practice of "empathy, forgiveness, love, and compassion" lead to a sense of sympathy and accountability? Perhaps a reflexive approach to deconstructing the silencing of racialized voices would lend arms to the embracing of unheard voices in the educational system.

Despite the recommendations of the Truth and Reconciliation Commission of Canada, Indigenous people continue to struggle from a system built on discrimination which perpetuates marginalization and inflicts pain. The bell now tolls for the instillers of knowledge to create spaces for students and faculty to engage in the discourse of re-engagement. The chapters in the book serve as doorways to conversations that can lead to healing and reconciliation. For example, in the part "Telling and Reliving Trauma as Pedagogy," chapters highlight the importance of risk-taking and shedding light on the oppressions that have existed. In the part titled "Pedagogies of Overcoming Silence," various approaches such as poetry, self-location, and auto-ethnography are provided as methodologies and access points to a pedagogy of pain and suffering. Finally, the part "Forgetting as Pedagogy" explores Indigenous women's healing, sacred ecology, bibliography, and poetry.

Overall, this book being the first of its kind, articulates the thought that sharing pain and suffering in an authentic way can be cathartic, therapeutic, and transformative. To achieve the desired goal, conversations must continue. The hope is that reflexivity and engagement will disrupt oppression in education and other contexts as a form of critical pedagogy as we continue to advocate for disruptive counternarratives.

Magnus Mfoafo-M'Carthy
Associate Professor
Wilfrid Laurier University

Contributors

Charis Auger ("Old Lady Bear That Beautifies Where She Walks in the Bush") embraces Elder's teachings and believes that *when you are gifted a story, you take care of that story. You nurture that story. You give away that story when someone needs it.* Auger lives this philosophy as a Two-Spirited Cree woman and creates spaces where Others who are silenced and marginalized feel safe in sharing their experiences. Auger is well-known for being a passionate social justice advocate. She has a deep respect for contributing to an inclusive Canada where all lives are valued – a community where everyone can join the conversation. Auger is an emerging scholar motivated to engage in research for social change, influencing governmental, institutional, and community-based diversity, equity, and inclusivity policies.

Christina Belcher is Emeritus Full Professor in Education at Redeemer University, Canada. Her research interests include higher education, children's literature, worldview, culture, technology, and the use of literature in disability studies. In addition, she is an unapologetic bookaholic, with an eclectic research appetite and enjoys working collaboratively.

Andrew B. Campbell (@DRABC14) is a graduate of the University of Toronto, Canada, with a PhD in educational leadership, policy, and diversity. He is presently Adjunct Assistant Professor at Queen's University, Canada, in the Professional Master of Education (PME) Online and a faculty member at the University of Toronto in the Master of Teaching (MT) programme in the Department of Curriculum Teaching and Learning (CTL). He is an Ontario Certified Teacher (OCT) and has taught at all levels of the education system for the last 25 years in Jamaica, Bahamas, and Canada. His research and teaching focus on issues of equity and inclusion, educational leadership, Black LGBTQ+ issues, teacher education, and teacher performance evaluation. You can learn more about DR. ABC and his work on his website DR. ABC (https://drabc.ca/).

Ardavan Eizadirad (@DrEizadirad) is Assistant Professor in the Faculty of Education at Wilfrid Laurier University, Canada; and an instructor in the Faculty of Social Work, Master of Teaching, and Bachelor of Education programme at the University of Toronto, Canada. He is an educator with the Toronto District School Board; author of *Decolonizing Educational Assessment: Ontario Elementary Students and the EQAO* (2019); and co-editor of *Equity as Praxis in Early Childhood Education and Care* (2021 co-edited with Zuhra Abawi and Rachel Berman) and *International Handbook of Anti-Discriminatory Education* (forthcoming 2023, co-edited with Peter Trifonas). Eizadirad is also the founder and director of EDIcation Consulting (www.edication.org) offering equity, diversity, and inclusion training to organizations. He is also a community activist with the non-profit organization Youth Association for Academics, Athletics, and Character Education (YAAACE) in the Jane and Finch community in Toronto; a board of directors member for Amadeusz, which provides educational programmes and services for incarcerated youth and young adults; and a member of the Race and Identity-Based Data Collection Community Advisory Panel with the Toronto Police Services. His research interests include equity, standardized testing, community engagement, anti-oppressive practices, critical pedagogy, social justice education, resistance, and decolonization.

Reginald K. Ellis specializes in the history of Historically Black Colleges and Universities (HBCUs) and African American leaders during the Jim Crow era. His first manuscript, titled *Between Washington and Du Bois: The Racial Politics of James Edward Shepard* (2017), is an analytical biography of James Edward Shepard, the founding president of North Carolina Central University, located in Durham, North Carolina. This work was published by the University Press of Florida. Ellis co-edited the anthology *The Seedtime: The Work and the Harvest: New Perspectives on the Black Freedom Struggle in America* (2018) with Jeffery Littlejohn and Peter Levey. A former National Endowment for the Humanities scholar (2013), Ellis was one of 30 scholars to serve as a fellow in the Summer Institute at Harvard University's Du Bois Institute on African American Struggles for Freedom and Civil Rights. Notwithstanding his scholarship, instruction, and administrative roles, Ellis has remained active with a number of organizations, including the Graduate Association for African American History (GAAAH), which currently hosts the African American History conference at the University of Memphis; the American Historical Association as a councilman in the Professional Division; and on the board of directors of the Florida Humanities Councils. Ellis is active in the community by participating in a number of capacities and is a member of Leadership Tallahassee Class 31, Leadership Florida Connect Class IX, and past member of the board of directors for the Legal Aid Foundation Tallahassee. Additionally, Ellis remains active in a host of professional and academic organizations, including the Gamma Mu Lambda Chapter of Alpha Phi Alpha Fraternity, Incorporated; the Association for the Study of African American Life and History (ASALH); the Southern Conference on African and African American Studies, Incorporated (SCAASI); the Organization of American Historians (OAH); and the Southern Historical Association (SHA).

Zahra Kasamali is Assistant Professor in the Department of Curriculum and Pedagogy at Brandon University, Canada. She is also Adjunct Professor in the Department of Secondary Education at the University of Alberta, Canada. She received her PhD in secondary education with a specialization in curriculum studies from the University of Alberta. Her scholarship interests include holistic education, wisdom traditions, intersectional approaches to education connected to spiritual sensibilities, Indigenous philosophies, pedagogical practices, and Sufic sensibilities.

Sundra D. Kincey is Assistant Vice President of Program Quality and SACSCOC Liaison at Florida A&M University (FAMU), USA, where she provides leadership in academic programme authorization, programme review, and specialized accreditation. She also serves as the champion and advocate of textbook affordability solutions for students at FAMU. Kincey's experiences expand more than 20 years in higher education at Historically Black Colleges and Universities, a predominantly white institution, and system-level office for public universities. Her research interests are the retention, persistence, and academic success of minority students.

Anita Lafferty is a PhD candidate at the University of Alberta, Canada, in the Faculty of Secondary Education. She is of Dene and Cree descent, and a member of the Líídlı̨ı̨ Kų́ę́ First Nation in the Northwest Territories, Canada. Her doctoral research examines approaches of Indigenous curriculum perspectives that are grounded in Dene k'ę́ę́ (philosophy) of the Land. Her research includes learning from/with the Land, experiences of Indigenous youth, identity, healing, and matriarchal knowledge. She takes a multidisciplinary approach in her research drawing on the fields of multi-media, art, poetry, storytelling, and Indigenous methodologies.

Daniel Lumsden is a secondary school teacher in Toronto, Canada, specializing in accounting and mathematics. He completed his undergraduate degrees in business administration (2000) and information systems (2001) at St. Francis Xavier University, Canada. Lumsden holds a BA of education (2003) and a MA in adult education (2006) from the Ontario Institute for Studies in Education (OISE) at the University of Toronto, and a MA of educational leadership (2021) from Memorial University of Newfoundland, Canada. He holds a PhD in education from OISE (2018) and is currently pursuing a MA in educational technology from the University of Michigan–Dearborn, USA. His dissertation research, examined teachers' perceptions on the use of video instruction in the flipped classroom, with a primary focus in secondary mathematics. Lumsden's research study interests are in flipped classrooms and anti-racist education. He has presented his research internationally and is a member of the Flipped Learning Global Initiative. Lumsden was also the president of the Canadian African Diaspora while he attended St. Francis Xavier University, Canada. He is also a member of the anti-racism committee at the school he currently teaches at, where he has presented workshops for faculty and staff, along with acquiring guest presenters that are already doing the work. Finally, Lumsden moderates an anti-racism book club with his faculty and staff members, where they meet once a month to discuss issues facing communities and how the books are addressing these experiences.

Kateri Marie Marandola is an Intermediate French Immersion teacher employed by the Niagara Catholic District School Board. She has been in the field of education for the past 16 years and resides in St. Catharines, Ontario, Canada, with her husband Michael and their 12-year-old son Mikah. Marandola was born and raised in the Northern Ontario city of Sault Ste. Marie where she began her post-secondary education at Algoma University, Canada, in 2000. After three years of study at Algoma University, Marandola transferred to Laurentian University, Canada. She received an honours BA degree in law and justice from Laurentian in 2004. She continued her education at Nipissing University, Canada, where she completed the BA of education programme in 2005. While working for the Niagara Catholic District School Board, Marandola completed a MA of education from Nipissing University. Her master's research, titled "Self-Location: An Indigenous Research Approach to Educational Development and Practice" focuses on the background and principal works of Indigenous education. The contents are an amalgamation of her master's research, as well as personal and professional community connections. Marandola was greatly influenced throughout her life by social justice issues and community work in Northern Ontario. Her life experiences with the community and her career in education has been the foundation and inspiration for her advocacy for educational reform. Marandola is a strong ally and advocate working in partnership within her school with the Indigenous community to bring awareness to educators and students about Indigenous history and culture. Her focus, through the practice of self-location, is to support the journey of healing relationships by making common connections, encouraging empathy through education, and developing strong and compassionate leaders for the future.

Julie A. Mooney is a Canadian settler of Irish-Scottish ancestry living and working in Treaty 6 territory and the Homeland of the Métis Nation.

She is a PhD candidate in educational policy studies at the University of Alberta, Canada, specializing in adult, community, and higher education. Her doctoral research uses narrative inquiry to explore how Canadian university professors are learning, in partnership with local Indigenous communities and with the support of educational developers, to implement institutional policies to indigenize and decolonize teaching and curricular practices.

Alicia Noreiga is a PhD candidate in the Faculty of Education at the University of New Brunswick, Canada. Noreiga is interested in studies that promote social justice and equity. Through her academic focus and advocacy, Noreiga hopes to raise awareness of, and assist in transforming, inequitable systems that disadvantage marginalized groups. As such, her research path includes critical participatory methodologies that amplify the voices of queer, Black, and rural communities.

Sharla Mskokii Peltier (Sharla Mskokii Kwe), a member of Mnjikaning (Rama) First Nation, Ontario, is an Assistant Professor in the Faculty of Education at University of Alberta, Canada. Her research and teaching experiences in community and post-secondary contexts are rich with storytelling, community land-based pedagogy, and relational teachings. Mskokii Kwe's scholarship centres Indigenous teaching-learning practices and Indigenous research methods.

Ameenah Shakir is Director of the Candidate Empowerment Center (CEC), Title III funded programme, and serves as the Living Learning Community liaison in the College of Education at Florida A&M University (FAMU), USA. Additionally, she teaches African American history courses in FAMU's History and Political Science Department and health activism courses in the Women's Study Program at Florida State University, USA. Shakir's research curates the ways in which African American women's professional endeavours challenged race, sex, and class discrimination. To this end, she is revising a book manuscript titled *Birthing Liberation: Dr. Helen Dickens and Health Activism in Post-War America*. She has presented at numerous academic conferences, served on national committees for granting agencies, facilitated administrator/faculty trainings for the African American History Taskforce, and is the recipient of several awards and honours including the McKnight Fellowship and the National Endowment for the Humanities Fellowship, and served as a C-SPAN Lecturer in History. ORCID: https://orcid.org/0000-0001-7086-7230

Steve Sider (@drstevesider) is a Professor in the Faculty of Education at Wilfrid Laurier University, Canada, where he teaches courses in international education, school leadership, and inclusive education. He is the past president of the Comparative and International Education Society of Canada and the current director of the Centre for Leading Research in Education, a university research centre exploring interdisciplinary aspects of education, He is the inaugural programme coordinator for the Laurier Bachelor of Arts in International Education Studies programme, the first of its kind in Canada. He is a fellow at the Balsillie School of International Affairs and an Associate of Inclusive Education Canada and the Canadian Research Centre on Inclusive Education. Sider currently holds three Canadian national research grants examining inclusive leadership practices of school principals in Canada, Haiti, and Ghana. Recent publications can be found on his research team website www .leadtoinclude.org. Prior to his work in the Faculty of Education, Sider was a school administrator, special education teacher, and classroom teacher for 15 years.

Jessica Vorstermans is an Assistant Professor in the critical disability studies programme in the School of Health Policy and Management, Faculty of Health at York University, Canada. Her research makes critical interventions into the field of international experiential and service learning and global citizenship, engaging plural ideas of human rights, disability, and equity in our current neoliberal world. She uses critical disability theory and the lens of intersectionality to complicate North–South encounters that produce impairment and disablement. Her ongoing work engages community-based research; centres the perspectives and desires of those in the South; and takes up equity and critical care in community, disability, and North/South relations.

Allyson L. Watson serves as a Dean for the College of Education at Florida A&M University, USA. Watson has focused her research on innovation in education, STEM in urban education, women and faculty of colour in higher education, and urban school and university partnerships. She is a full professor and tenured graduate faculty with substantial teaching and research experience in educational research, advanced educational measurements and statistics, public school relations, and instructional strategies. Watson spent over 20 years teaching and leading in Tulsa, Oklahoma. Her work in north Tulsa shaped her passion for encouraging teachers to include accurate history within culturally responsive pedagogy.

Darius J. Young is a native of Detroit, Michigan, and a two-time graduate of Florida A&M University, USA. In 2011, Young completed his PhD in 20th century U.S. history from the University of Memphis, USA. He is an author and historian of Black political movements during the 20th century. His first book, *Robert R. Church Jr. and the African American Political Struggle* (2019), won the C. Calvin Smith Book Award from the Southern Conference on African American Studies, Incorporated. His current project, *Freedom Now!: Albert B. Cleage Jr. and the Black Power Movement in Detroit,* will examine the life and activism of the founder of Black Liberation Theology, Albert Cleage Jr. Young has published a series of articles, book chapters, and reviews that can be found in the African American Intellectual History Society's *Black Perspectives*, *The Journal of African American History*, *The Journal of Southern History*, *The Journal of American History*, *The Griot: The Journal of African American Studies*, and the *Florida Historical Quarterly*. Young is the recipient of several awards including the Southern Regional Education Board Doctoral Scholars Fellowship, the Gilder Lehrman Institute of American History Research Fellowship, and the Benjamin L. Hooks Institute for Social Change Teaching Fellowship. He is the recipient of the Florida A&M Center for Disability Access and Research Faculty Pacesetter Award (2012), the Florida A&M Teacher of the Year Award (2013), the Florida A&M Advanced Teacher of the Year Award (2018), and the Southern Conference on African American Studies Member of the Year (2019). He is a member of the Association for the Study of African American Life and History; Southern Conference on African American Studies, Inc.; the American Studies Association; Organization of American Historians; and Alpha Phi Alpha Fraternity, Incorporated.

1 Centring Pedagogies of Pain and Suffering by Embracing Our Wounds and Scars

Ardavan Eizadirad, Andrew B. Campbell, and Steve Sider

We began planning for this book in 2020 after we received a high number of article submissions for a special issue of the journal *Diaspora, Indigenous, and Minority Education* (https://www.tandfonline.com/action/journalInformation?show=aimsScope&journalCode=hdim20) with the title "Visibilizing Systemic Wounds of Oppression in Education via Pedagogy of Engaging with Pain & Suffering." From the submissions, it was evident that there was a strong interest in engaging in this work. Therefore, we began exploring multiple platforms to create dialogue and conversations about pedagogies of engaging pain and suffering. The special issue of *Diaspora, Indigenous, and Minority Education* was published in September 2021, and this book supplements the themes in the issue, which is the first of its kind!

We begin this chapter by discussing how the idea for this book further developed based on formal and informal conversations about willing to be uncomfortable by opening up about our vulnerabilities, including past and present experiences of pain, suffering, and trauma. Next, our positionalities as co-editors are outlined in terms of our identities, and lived and professional experiences. As part of creating a brave space with readers, we also share personal things that you may not know about us. We encourage you to reflect on your own life and experiences to begin constructively engaging with your own pain, suffering, and trauma. Building on this, the chapter then situates the collective work in this book by providing an overview of the three themes (parts), which demonstrate pedagogies of pain and suffering in various contexts, and their impact as therapeutic and transformative as a form of critical pedagogy. We make the argument that the language of pain and suffering is universal, hence its potential as a medium and pedagogy for transformative teaching and learning.

Overall, the book builds on key aspects of critical pedagogy (Freire, 1970; Grioux & McLaren, 1989; Ladson-Billings, 1995; Noddings, 2013) across different contexts identifying the process of engaging with pain and suffering, and sharing it with others as therapeutic and transformative. This can offer both personal and systemic liberation. Engaging with pedagogies of pain and suffering is timely given that representations of oppression, often captured via images and videos and shared on social

DOI: 10.4324/9781003205296-1

media platforms and news outlets, are hypervisibilized as part of discussions about inequitable practices within educational institutions. Recent examples would be the public trial of the police officer for the murder of George Floyd in the United States and the discovery of more than 5,000 and counting unmarked grave sites of Indigenous children in various parts of Canada.

This edited volume is a synthesis of storytelling about pain and trauma and the act of telling, narrating, and sharing experiences with intentionality as a form of critical pedagogy. It is important to discuss both the act of narrating and how it is told as a pedagogy to simultaneously understand the complexities and nuances involved in its processes, hence the potential for transformative change both for the narrator and the audience. Engaging with (re)telling of pain and suffering involves revisiting traumatic experiences which can evoke a range of emotions including anger, sadness, anxiety, and frustration amongst many others emotions and feelings. Yet, as Audre Lorde (2017) reminds us:

> But anger expressed and translated into action in the service of our vision and our future is a liberating and strengthening act of clarification, for it is in the painful process of this translation that we identify who are our allies with whom we have grave differences, and who are our genuine enemies. Anger is loaded with information and energy.
>
> (p. 23)

The act of storytelling as a medium allows for the harnessing of negative emotions and feelings to inform intentional pedagogy. This is a dialogical process (Freire, 1970; Ennser-Kananen, 2016) which impacts the narrator by opening up and sharing painful experiences, while simultaneously impacting the audience based on what is told, how it is told, and through what medium. As hooks (2000) points out:

> [T]he place of suffering – the place where we are broken in spirit, when accepted and embraced, is also a place of peace and possibility. Our sufferings do not magically end; instead we are able to wisely alchemically recycle them. They become the abundant waste that we use to make new growth possible … Learning to embrace our suffering is one of the gifts offered by spiritual life and practice. (pp. 80–81)

Hence, on one level this book is about centring marginalized voices, sharing their experiences of pain and oppression, and on another level, emphasizing how their stories are told with intentionality, "alchemically recycled," to learn, unlearn, and disrupt normalizing practices that have and continue to enact harm in education.

A Framework for Engaging with Pain and Suffering as Critical Pedagogy

The collection of chapters in this volume draws on diverse experiences, auto-ethnographies, and case studies situated in a number of intersecting theoretical and methodological frameworks, including culturally sustaining pedagogy (Paris, 2012), lived experience and hermeneutic phenomenology (van Manen, 2017), and narrative inquiry and autoethnography (Clandinin, 2016) to showcase non-hegemonic ways of engaging pain and suffering as critical pedagogy. As the co-editors, through multiple meetings and ongoing discussions, we have outlined three themes serving as parts of the book. The three themes are:

1) Telling and reliving trauma as pedagogy.
2) Pedagogies of overcoming silence.
3) Forgetting pedagogy.

These themes are further explained in detail at the start of each part of the book. The themes as a collective serve as a framework for the different ways we can engage with pain and suffering. These pedagogies are not exclusive in nature nor do they operate in silos. A typical trajectory could be going from forgetting to overcoming silence and finally telling and sharing your trauma with intentionality, but there are multiple ways people can process trauma and this involves entry from various points and stages. There is no prescribed trajectory. How we have deconstructed these pedagogies, and in what order, is one way to map them amongst many other possible trajectories.

We invite you as the reader to find yourself and your story in the midst of your pain and trauma. Even institutions have tried to regulate how pain and suffering should be shared, in what spaces, and through what mediums. Although we have placed the various chapters in this book within a theme, the experiences discussed by the authors overlap across the themes from different angles and to varying degrees. Rather, the themes are outlined to help us theorize critical pedagogy and to advance concepts related to engaging with pain and suffering. For example, tears, blood, and sweat can symbolize emotions for different occasions ranging from joy and happiness to sadness and anger. Therefore, context matters! Also, we experience emotions individually and as a collective impacted by power dynamics within spaces. Hence, the three themes provide a framework to help readers contextualize and understand the pain and suffering outlined by the authors, while also making connections to our collective humanity. As Lorde (1984) eloquently put it, "There is no such thing as a single issue struggle because we do not lead single issue lives" (p. 147).

By centring lived experiences of racialized and minoritized identities as counternarratives, the book identifies and challenges systemic forms of oppression and inequities across multiple contexts in education which continue to dehumanize individuals and social groups in relation to normalized ideas, policies, and institutional practices. Chapter contributors share personal and collective experiences of pain and suffering with others as a therapeutic, instructive, and powerfully transformative process. Chapters further foreground narratives which represent non-dominant forms of knowledge and lived experiences in education, historically dismissed as "less valuable."

We argue that the act of telling, narrating, or sharing experiences of pain and suffering is a pedagogy in its own right. Ennser-Kananen (2016) offers three ways in which pain can serve as pedagogy: becoming vulnerable while planning painful lessons, maintaining painful conversations, and promoting transformation (pp. 561–562). Similarly, this book emphasizes transformation through narration. As Iaquinta (2019) emphasizes:

> The commitment of pedagogy, and specifically of a pedagogy of pain, is therefore to recognize and accept the dimension of pain in the educational experience and imagine, hypothesize, build, modalities and practices that allow the subject to give name and voice to the pain to go through it. (p. 106)

Overall, this book explores processes of narrating pain and how pain is shared pedagogically. This means being conscious of who is doing the narrating, to whom, and for what purposes. As a collective, the chapters seek to shift the conversations towards understanding inequities in education on a systemic level, where hierarchical power relations often discourage dissent, dismiss stories of suffering as exceptions, and mute narratives of oppression told by racialized and minoritized voices (Abawi et al., 2021; Eizadirad & Campbell, 2021; hooks, 2003; Matias, 2013; Truth and Reconciliation Commission of Canada, 2015). In centring counternarratives, as part of accepting chapters for this volume, author positionalities were assessed to ensure representation in terms of identity, lived and professional experiences, and the range of issues discussed. Chapters include contributions from scholars, community activists, practitioners, and graduate students who offer powerful illustrations of the way in which narratives of pain and suffering can be transformed into valuable teachable opportunities. This, in turn, can challenge inequitable and unjust educational policies and practices that have historically been normalized and often unquestioned.

Trust and Calculated Risk-Taking in Embracing Vulnerabilities

Trust is essential in cultivating brave spaces that promote socio-emotional intelligence and sharing of vulnerabilities with others. How often do we conform as scholars and educators to amplify our professional duties and experiences at the expense of marginalizing our lived experiences and vulnerabilities? We are often told by educational institutions that only selective spaces are appropriate for expression of emotions and vulnerabilities. Why is this? Which institutional policies, practices, and processes have contributed to perpetuating this as the norm? Who is going to share their pain and vulnerabilities as part of their professional profile and for what purposes? We highly encourage you to start doing this as educators! As Miller (2018) explains in his book *Love and Compassion: Exploring Their Role in Education*, "By accepting pain in ourselves, we learn to be present to pain in others" (p. 131). Hopefully, by the end of reading this book we have convinced you as a reader of the benefits of this approach and as a key component of engaging pain and suffering constructively.

As co-editors we have learned to become comfortable in our vulnerable experiences as a means to build trust and grow as a collective, because "[t]he inability to connect with others carries with it an inability to assume responsibility for causing pain" (hooks, 2000, p. 39). As individuals with different identities from walks of life across various geographical locations, including Iran, India, and Jamaica, with varying lived and professional experiences, we took time to learn about one another beyond our academic duties. This involved being honest with ourselves and each other. We started all meetings planning this book with life check-ins where we shared the highs, lows, and ugly experiences we were going through. Whereas often we supported one another, there were also times when we disagreed and made each other upset and angry. Yet, the trust we built by willing to be vulnerable and openly share our pain and suffering was foundational in allowing us to work through the negative emotions to advance our larger goal of challenging inequities and social injustices in education. Trust allows for vulnerabilities to be shared. The vulnerability allows for more of the authentic self to be expressed. The more we express our authentic self allows for opportunities for transformative teaching and learning.

Disrupting oppression in educational contexts also involves calculated risk-taking where one chooses to be brave in the face of fears and anxieties (Donald, 2013; Eizadirad & Portelli, 2018; Hanna, 2019). As Albert Woodfox (2019), a Black man who spent 40 years in solitary confinement in the United States, shares in his autobiography titled *Solitary: Unbroken by Four Decades in Solitary Confinement. My Story of Transformation and Hope*, "[C]ourage doesn't mean that you aren't afraid. Courage means that you master that fear and act in spite of being afraid" (p. 15). Therefore, it is not that fear or anxiety is non-existent, but we have built consciousness, coping mechanisms, support networks, and strategies to work through such negative emotions to advance critical pedagogy. This is different from the #OppressionOlympics that often equity and social justice conversations shift towards when people share their vulnerabilities in justifying who has experienced more oppression. In turn, when conversations go in that direction, it takes away from challenging the root causes of oppressive practices embedded within institutional policies and practices.

Often institutions want to regulate how, when, and where we share our emotions (Hanna, 2019). As co-editors, we choose to be a living embodiment of a counternarrative from our physical presence to how we demonstrate and share our beliefs, values, and lived experiences with others via implementation of certain practices. With intentionality we challenge the normalized neoliberal model of education that has made schooling all about what kinds of jobs you can get, instead of education being about personal and transformative growth. The power of willing to be vulnerable and intentional in self-disclosure is a form of strength and resiliency in disrupting oppression within educational institutions. We model this next in how we share our narratives to cultivate trust with colleagues, students, and you as the reader with the goal of advancing equitable outcomes and centring social justice in who we are, how we live, and how we enact our pedagogies.

Sharing Our Authentic Selves as Counternarratives

As a starting point and a reflective exercise, we share with you the readers our professional biographies shared on university affiliated websites that emphasize our scholarly work, research grants, and publications. We have supplemented these biographies with a paragraph stating "But here is what you may not know about …" where we outline our other lived experiences and passions so you can learn more about our authentic selves rooted in vulnerabilities we have experienced. This serves as a counternarrative to the hegemonic practice where educational institutions emphasize and outline academic work in assessing "worth" of scholars measured by how much is published and how fast (Brown & Strega, 2005). This practice is normalized and legitimized as standard practice in many post-secondary educational institutions where professors and faculty are required to submit annual currency reports to outline their growth and involvement with publications and conferences. This has become a compulsory component in the trajectory of becoming a tenured professor. Who does this process privilege and who does it oppress? What is neglected when this process becomes the norm? Whose needs does it oppress at the individual and community level?

Dr. Ardavan Eizadirad (@DrEizadirad) is an Assistant Professor in the Faculty of Education at Wilfrid Laurier University; and an instructor in the School of Early Childhood Studies at Ryerson University, and in the Faculty of Social Work, Master of Teaching, and Bachelor of Education programme at University of Toronto. He is an educator with the Toronto District School Board, author of *Decolonizing Educational Assessment: Ontario Elementary Students and the EQAO* (2019), and co-editor of *Equity as Praxis in Early Childhood Education and Care* (2021), and *International Handbook of Anti-Discriminatory Education* (forthcoming 2023). His research interests include equity, standardized testing, community engagement, anti-oppressive practices, critical pedagogy, social justice education, resistance, and decolonization.

But here is what you may not know about Ardavan: I immigrated from Iran to Canada in 1998 with my family as an English as a second language learner. When the plane landed in Toronto on a cold day in October, it was the first time I saw snow. My grandfather spent time in jail in Iran as a political prisoner. My grandmother died when I was a teenager and I did not handle it well, as it was the first time I had to deal with death on an intimate level. My mother is a social worker helping newly immigrants resettle in Toronto, Canada. My father is an agricultural engineer who could not find work in his field upon arrival in Canada due to systemic barriers, and hence settled for being a courier driver to support our family. I have officiated basketball as a referee for 16 years and am currently an international basketball official for wheelchair basketball. I love poetry and spoken word, particularly the works of Rumi, Hafez, and Taalam Acey. My favourite foods are kabobs, chicken wings, and Torshi Tareh, which is a traditional stew dish with origins from the north of Iran. I have two tattoos. The first one is located on my right arm and it is a picture of praying hands with a ribbon going around it stating "In Loving Memory of Grandma" (Figure 1.1).

My other tattoo is located on the right side of my ribs and written in Persian calligraphy turned into art which states "Through love thorns become roses" (Figure 1.2).

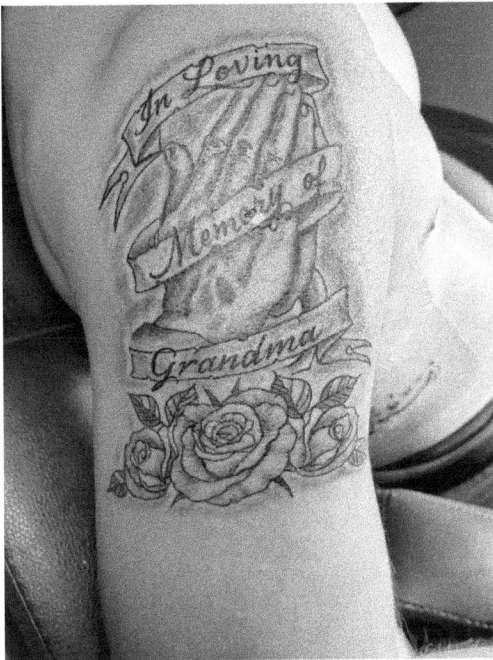

Figure 1.1 Ardavan's arm tattoo expressing "In Loving Memory of Grandma."

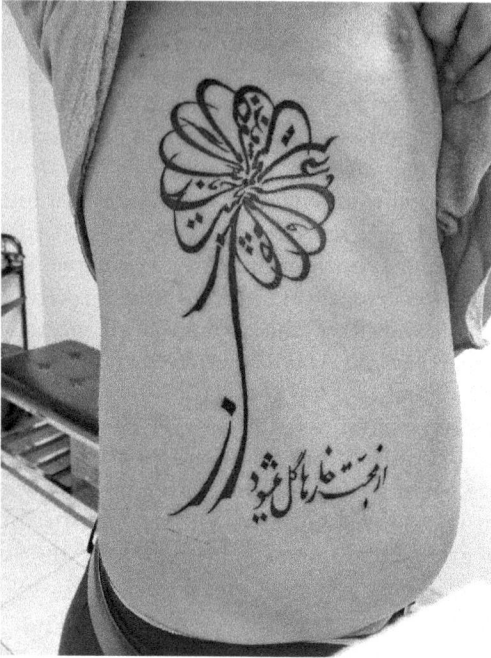

Figure 1.2 Ardavan's rib tattoo in Persian calligraphy expressing "Through love thorns become roses."

Tattoos were a medium at critical times in my life to constructively express the negative emotions and feelings I was experiencing. I am also the founder of EDIcation Consulting (www.edication.org) offering equity, diversity, and inclusion training to organizations. I am also a community activist being involved with the non-profit organizations Youth Association for Academics, Athletics, and Character Education (YAAACE) in the Jane and Finch community (http://yaaace.com/); a board of directors member for Amadeusz (http://amadeusz.ca/), which provides educational programmes and services for incarcerated youth and young adults; and a member of the Toronto Police Services' Race and Identity-Based Data Collection Community Advisory Panel. Do you look at me differently now?

Dr. Andrew B. Campbell (@DRABC14) is a graduate of the University of Toronto, with a PhD in educational leadership, policy, and diversity. He is presently an Adjunct Assistant Professor at Queen's University in the Professional Master of Education (PME) Online and a faculty member at the University of Toronto, in the Master of Teaching (MT) programme, in the Department of Curriculum Teaching and Learning (CTL). He is an Ontario Certified Teacher (OCT) and has taught at all levels of the education system for the last 25 years, in Jamaica, Bahamas, and Canada. His research and teaching focus on issues of equity and inclusion, educational leadership, Black LGBTQ+ issues, teacher education, and teacher performance evaluation.

But here is what you may not know about Andrew: In preparing to write this section of the chapter, I thought long and hard about which part of me I should share and which wound, pain, or scars would be most "appropriate" to share in a book like this. After many discussions about the formatting of the chapter, I still engaged myself in another discussion on the rationale and purpose of showing a wound or scar. In that moment, I was reminded of the power and impact of my storytelling. I choose to share a few excerpts from my book *The Invisible Student in the Jamaican Classroom* (2018).

I walk into all rooms as a six feet, four inches tall Black man who is confident, bold, and intentional. This is seen in my walk, fashion, conversation, and interaction with anyone in the space. However, it was not always like that. For years, I was an invisible student. For years I was made invisible by a school system that I did not feel a sense of belonging to. Instead, many days I dreaded school, I was scared of the classroom, scared of being left alone with students who would hurt me. For many of those years, I also chose to be invisible at times. That invisibility was a shield and protection, "if they don't see me, then they can't hurt me" was what I would tell myself.

> I know what it is to attend school in Jamaica and experience formal schooling as a child being bullied with every level of name-calling you could think of, being questioned by students and teachers alike, being reprimanded for my effeminate behaviour and being reminded to be a man!
>
> (p. 7)

In sharing the not so known parts of my story, past pain, present scars, I am reminded that many readers may still be suffering from the inability to share and embrace their wounds. This is the reason why I've been sharing my past trauma in my storytelling.

> Years ago, I wished I had a classroom teacher, a guidance counsellor, or a Sunday school teacher to tell how much I was hurting and how much I was scared. I wish I had someone to tell the boys to stop calling me names. I wish I had someone who would tell me it was okay to not like football. I wish I had someone who encouraged me to follow my passion for dancing. (p. 9)

He is invisible because he does not wish to be seen. He is invisible because he knows he has not been seen by those who he wishes to be seen by. He is invisible because he is disengaged from school – present physically most of the time but emotional and socially absent … The feeling of invisibility is something that many LGBT people experience. This is especially problematic in our Jamaican context where visibility is risky. Our young gay men do not have many local role models and are constantly bombarded with negative stereotypical images of the gay male. It is very difficult when there are hardly any positive images like you around. ... feeling inadequate, feeling less than, and being too frightened and too scared. So, they become anything else but themselves and constantly fight to remain invisible. Being invisible is a safe space. (p. 15)

When I was young, I did not see any gay role models, except for those on TV. I did not see the successful, black, gay man that would have given me the courage and hope to know that I can become more than what the schools and neighbourhood bullies said I would become. So, this level of disclosure is important and necessary for this work. (p. 9)

I am one of those who have proven the power and impact that this retelling can have on others. I tell my story, not to listen to my voice or wallow in the pain for attention, but because I know the healing and transformative power in sharing that, inviting the listeners to be inspired and moved to share their own stories, and in doing so, experience the same release that I have had, and gaining the same power and joy that I now possess.

I want to remind scholars as you do the work within the space of equity and social justice – being in tune with who you are, understanding how your lived experiences impact your positionality – to value the power of your own story, even those parts that the institutions consider unimportant.

I, therefore, thought it important to not only gather external voices and share their lived experiences, but also to ensure that my voice and my story was captured as an example of my advocacy, my truth, my own coming out, and my celebration. (p. 7)

Dr. Steve Sider (@DrSteveSider) is Professor in the Faculty of Education at Wilfrid Laurier University in Waterloo, Canada. He is the past president of the Comparative and International Education Society of Canada. He currently holds three Canadian national research grants examining inclusive leadership practices of Canadian school principals. Recent publications have included a co-edited book which provides comparative and international perspectives on education as well as articles in *International Studies in Educational Administration*, *Canadian Journal of Education*, and *Comparative and International Education*. He is the inaugural programme coordinator for the Bachelor of Arts in International Education Studies programme, the first of its kind in Canada. He is the director of the Centre for Leading Research in Education. Prior to his work in the Faculty of Education, Sider was a school administrator, special education teacher, and classroom teacher for 15 years.

But here is what you may not know about Steve: I grew up in northeast India, the child of Canadian parents who had moved to India to be involved in community development work. I had my early schooling in the local community and in a boarding school a 24-hour train ride away from home. At the age of eight, my family returned to Canada, a country that was completely foreign to me. I completed my schooling in Canada (even as I write this, a few words cannot encapsulate the challenges that went with this experience ... the pain of not knowing anyone, of being bullied, of language and learning difficulties, of poor health), eventually completing post-secondary education and becoming a secondary school teacher.

I taught courses on world history and global economics. For a portion of this time, I taught in an international school with students from around the world. I led experiential learning opportunities for my students, travelling with them to countries such as Thailand, Venezuela, and France. I thoroughly enjoyed the process of helping my students develop a broader perspective on the world. I pursued graduate studies while I was a teacher and school administrator, partly just because I loved to learn. Although I had been a teacher who was committed to global education and perspective building, I did not yet know about the formal scholarship of comparative and international education until completing my PhD.

As I have engaged in comparative and international education research, I have increasingly recognized the substantial privileges that I have experienced. My lived experience has been framed by my cultural and racial background as a white person, the child of development workers, and growing up in northern Bihar, an area of India that is considered one of the poorest in the country. As a child, I spoke Hindi as my first language. I soon recognized the power of the English language as a result of an American boarding school experience. The school, nestled in the Himalayan foothills, connected me with children from around the world but separated me from the community that I considered home. Later, I was privileged through the support I received from school teachers who helped me transition to Canada; I recognize that not every child has these benefits. As a teacher, I was able to travel with students who were also privileged to have families who had the economic ability to support travel. The list of my privileges is substantial. I have lived in the tension of the guilt that goes along with these privileges and the acknowledgement that access to these privileges does not absolve me from trying to understand what it means to live in community and to work for justice within these communities. One thing that I have learned about education and myself is that there are lots of tensions and complexities in school and in life, and my own lived experience is representative of this. Do you look at me differently now?

Overall, as readers, we encourage you to pause and take a moment to reflect on your own life including your lived and professional experiences. Particularly, think about events that stirred up strong emotions and feelings in you and drastically impacted your life trajectory. If mapping this by writing it out, jotting notes, drawing, or other creative expressions aligns with your approach to learning, we encourage you to do this. Here are a series of questions to guide your reflection:

- If you had the luxury and opportunity to share some of your vulnerabilities, what would you share?
- Who would you share them with and why?
- What do these vulnerabilities represent?
- Why have you not shared them up to this point?
- What value can you find in sharing these vulnerabilities?
- How can sharing your pain and suffering be used as a form of critical pedagogy to build trust, sustain relationships with others, and cultivate a community of learners?

We highly suggest working through these questions at your own pace in conjunction with the vulnerabilities shared throughout the chapters by the various authors. We conclude by emphasizing that the language of pain and suffering is universal, and it is a starting point and a medium for coalition building to challenge systemic injustices and inequities.

References

Abawi, Z., Eizadirad, A., & Berman, R. (2021). *Equity as praxis in early childhood education and care*. Canadian Scholars Press.

Brown, L. A., & Strega, S. (2005). *Research as resistance: Critical, indigenous and anti-oppressive approaches*. Canadian Scholars' Press.

Campbell, A. B. (2018). The invisible student in the Jamaican classroom. USA. CreateSpace.

Clandinin, D. J. (2016). *Engaging in narrative inquiry*. Routledge

Donald, D. (2013). On making love to death: Plains Cree and Blackfoot wisdom. In M. Smith (Ed.), *Transforming the academy: Essays on indigenous education, knowledges and relations* (pp. 14–19). Canadian Federation for the Humanities and Social Sciences

Eizadirad, A., & Campbell, A. (2021). Visibilizing our pain and wounds as resistance and activist pedagogy to heal and hope: Reflections of 2 racialized professors. *Diaspora, Indigenous, and Minority Education*. https://doi.org/10.1080/15595692.2021.1937600

Eizadirad, A., & Portelli, J. (2018). Subversion in education: Common misunderstandings and myths. *International Journal of Critical Pedagogy*, 9(1), 53–72.

Ensser-Kananen, J. (2016). A pedagogy of pain: New directions for world language education. *The Modern Language Journal*, 100(2), 556–564. https://doi.org/10.1111/modl.1_12337

Freire, P. (1970). *Pedagogy of the oppressed*. The Continuum International Publishing Group Inc.

Giroux, H. A., McLaren, P. L., McLaren, P., & Peter, M. (Eds.). (1989). *Critical pedagogy, the state, and cultural struggle*. Suny Press.Chicago

Hanna, K. B. (2019). Pedagogies in the flesh: Building an anti-racist decolonized classroom. *Frontiers: A Journal of Women Studies, 40*(1), 229–244.

hooks, b. (2000). *All about love: New visions*. Harper Perennial.

hooks, b. (2003). *Teaching community: A pedagogy of hope*. Routledge.

Iaquinta, T. (2019). Education, person, suffering. Reflections of pain pedagogy. *European Journal of Education, 2*(2), 101–107.

Ladson-Billings, G. (1995). Toward a theory of culturally relevant pedagogy. *American Educational Research Journal, 32*(3), 465–491.

Lorde, A. (1984). *Learning from the 60s. Sister outsider: Essays and speeches*. Ten Speed Press.

Lorde, A. (2017). *The master's tools will never dismantle the master's house*. Penguin Random House UK.

Matias, C. E. (2013). Tears worth telling: Urban teaching and the possibilities of racial justice. *Multicultural Perspectives, 15*(4), 187–193.

Miller, J. P. (2018). *Love and compassion: Exploring their role in education*. University of Toronto Press.

Noddings, N. (2013). *Caring: A relational approach to ethics and moral education*. Univ of California Press.

Paris, D. (2012). Culturally sustaining pedagogy: A needed change in stance, terminology, and practice. *Educational Researcher, 41*(3), 93–97.

Truth and Reconciliation Commission of Canada. (2015). Truth and Reconciliation Commission of Canada: Calls to action. Retrieved from https://nctr.ca/assets/reports/Calls_to_Action_English2.pdf

Van Manen, M. (2017). Phenomenology and meaning attribution. *Indo-Pacific Journal of Phenomenology*. 17(1), 1–12. DOI: 10.1080/20797222.2017.1368253

Woodfox, A. (2019). *Solitary: Unbroken by four decades in solitary confinement. My story of transformation and hope*. Harper Collins.

Part 1

Telling and Reliving Trauma as Pedagogy

Until the lion learns to write, every story will glorify the hunter.

African Proverb

In a world dominated by historical and contemporary deficit and oppressive narratives, telling our stories and providing counternarratives is a bold and brave process that needs to be encouraged, particularly in spaces commonly occupied by racialized, marginalized, and historically oppressed and disenfranchised groups. Gatekeepers in dominant positions of power have set standards of how stories are to be told, what they should look like, and whose voices should be highlighted in academic spaces. Many of us have simply followed yet another set of prescribed behaviours for us. It is time more of us invoke and value the gift of storytelling we have held for generations, and disrupt the rules and norms meant not to uplift and promote us but to oppress and deny. One of those false myths that many have accepted is that telling a story of trauma and pain is damaging and presents the storyteller as weak. Furthermore, the norm has become that in academic spaces, we must present ourselves as capable, resolute, accomplished, and always striving to win. These are the very ideas that we seek to disrupt in this first part of the book. We want to ensure that readers understand the power in their stories if used effectively, timely, and strategically. That telling has the power to affirm, inspire, create, rescue, and heal.

Years ago in Jamaica during my undergraduate studies I (Andrew B. Campbell) did a course on counselling psychology with the last unit about who counsels the counsellor. It left a lasting impact on me. One of the main elements in the process of self-healing was the ability and skill in knowing how, when, and in what proportions to self-disclose. It was then that I understood the value of telling your story – stories that may be painful to share and painful to hear, but were necessary in the healing journey. There is something powerful in having the ability to share your story. For me, storytelling is a major counternarrative. Storytelling is something valuable and important for the survival of cultures and sustaining of communities. My African ancestors were not only able to preserve a culture that was forbidden by their colonial masters, but also able to transfer that culture

DOI: 10.4324/9781003205296-2

intergenerationally through storytelling and its multiple ways of knowing and being. In academia, there is much talk about sharing your lived experiences, bringing your authentic self to the teaching–learning dynamic, and allowing your students to get to know you. However, we can observe that these very desired outcomes have not been given equitable consideration and "permission" within academia. Whose stories are being told? Who gets access to tell their stories? When some of us who are Black, Indigenous, and racialized gain a voice and platform to tell our stories, the requests often come with specific parameters. Oftentimes, the stories requested are those that would force us to relive trauma and pain. Stories that many Black, Indigenous, racialized, equity-deserving scholars would rather not share – stories that many have not ventured into sharing and have not gained a handle on how to share.

Relationships are a key aspect of how you tell your story and for what purposes. What does it mean to be authentic and #KeepItReal? Is your story connected to hope and healing? Will your story inspire, motivate, and influence change? Will your story leave the audience agitated and triggered without adequate tools and support to gain and engage in the power of the story? These are some guiding questions to consider when making decisions about when, where, and how to tell your story. Storytelling is a vehicle for building relationships and having brave conversations that can work towards understanding and doing the work of transformative change. Storytelling should not be about #traumaPorn where it serves as a spectacle for entertainment and shock value. Instead, it is about intentional sharing as a form of critical pedagogy.

It takes bravery and a sense of safety to tell and relive. I find that most of us will share more of ourselves when we build trust and relationships with those around us, with those who listen to our stories, and with those who we trust with our stories. I often think of the privilege and responsibility I hold when students, colleagues, and community members trust me enough to retell and relive certain trauma in their lives. More often they do not require advice. What they require is a brave space to share and to open that trauma for the purpose of healing. They get it out in a space that is engulfed with trust, connections, and relationships. Telling and reliving trauma in spaces that lack trust, support, and caring relationships is unhealthy, dangerous, and harmful. There is no bravery or win in allowing others to be entertained by your trauma.

I wish to pause at this time and ensure I emphasize to the readers that storytelling is an art. Telling your stories is a skill to be developed over time. Telling and reliving trauma as pedagogy takes the same, or even more, investment in planning and preparation. We can further damage ourselves each time we share stories of trauma if we have not invested in intentional healing. Telling and reliving trauma is not for entertainment. Each time you tell such a story you share inner parts that belong to you. How do we then ensure that those listening walk away with the intentions behind your storytelling? Talking about trauma is not relieving the trauma for me. It is getting it out. I have had many opportunities to share stories about my experiences growing up in Jamaica, navigating oppressive spaces based on various parts of my identity, or dealing with course-related issues. In each of these storytelling episodes, I remember the feeling of "letting it out, letting it go" that I had. Telling about these was not only therapeutic and healing for me, but it was a lesson for my audience. Telling also gives you a gauge of your personal healing. There are stories that were told five years ago that were hard to tell; today they are easier. There are also other stories that are still hard to tell. Healing is a process; storytelling is a process.

I also model this in my classes and workshops. My teacher candidates get to see storytelling as impactful. They too have their stories. They too have broken parts that need healing and wholeness. They too can learn how to tell stories and heal. I have noticed the change in my students' listening patterns over the past three years. They are seeing the value of stories. They are being exposed to more racialized, Black, and Indigenous scholars, and to other ways of knowing and pedagogies.

2 Cultivating Brave Spaces to Take Risks to Challenge Systemic Oppression

*Andrew B. Campbell and
Ardavan Eizadirad*

Introduction: There Are No Safe Spaces!

This chapter is written by two racialized professors: Andrew who is Jamaican-Canadian and Ardavan who is Iranian-Canadian. Reflecting and sharing our identities and experiences via duoethnography and from a critical race theory (CRT) paradigm, we argue that there is no such thing as a safe space. We outline and theorize brave spaces (Arao & Clemens, 2013; Gilmour, 2021; Herrmann, 2017; Verduzco-Baker, 2018) as a counternarrative to safe spaces to facilitate unlearning and promote risk-taking to challenge systemic oppression. This aligns with what Micky Scottbey Jones (n.d.) outlines as key characteristics of brave spaces in her poem titled "An Invitation to a Brave Space":

An Invitation to a Brave Space

Listen
Together we will create brave space.
Because there is no such thing as a "safe space" –
We exist in the real world.
We all carry scars and we have all caused wounds.
In this space
We seek to turn down the volume of the outside world,
We amplify voices that fight to be heard elsewhere,
We call each other to more truth and love.
We have the right to start somewhere and continue to grow.
We have the responsibility to examine what we think we know.
We will not be perfect.
This space will not be perfect.
It will not always be what we wish it to be.
But
It will be our brave space together,
and
We will work on it side by side.

DOI: 10.4324/9781003205296-3

As conveyed in the language of the poem, brave spaces encourage stepping outside of comfort bubbles via calculated risk-taking and sharing and embracing of vulnerabilities. Within brave spaces, storytelling is enacted as critical pedagogy to share pain, suffering, and trauma to disrupt the norm with intentionality (Eizadirad & Campbell, 2021). Yet, it is not all roses and smooth sailing. Although brave spaces encourage authentic raw conversations and truth-telling from multiple perspectives, it also involves navigating tensions, drama, and unexpected teachable moments rooted in differences in opinions and lived experiences (Bourdieu, 1999; Freire, 1970). This is why it takes time to cultivate brave spaces with intentionality guided by love, respect, support, risk-taking, and reciprocity to foster trust and relationships to deconstruct tensions and harness collective action from the emotions expressed. As Bourdieu (1999) points out, "we must work with the multiple perspectives that correspond to the multiplicity of co-existing, and sometimes directly competing, points of view" (p. 3) as a means of arriving at new understanding and mobilizing as a collective.

It is important to recognize that not everyone is ready to share and converse about social issues that impact them, or express their pain and trauma in terms set by educators. We have to provide time and space for students to heal at their own pace. For example, there may be a shooting near the campus or in the neighbourhood, but this does not mean everyone wants to talk about it or is ready to discuss the shooting, including the impact of the event on their lives physically, socially, spiritually, or emotionally. It is good to create the space to discuss socioculturally relevant issues but also provide the option for people to pass and not engage in the topic if they are not ready and not view it as disengagement. As Gilmour (2021) explains, "It is common to hear the words 'safe space' in schools … [as] students need to feel physically safe, unafraid, and emotionally connected to learn," (p. 3), but just because educators declare that "this is a safe space," it does not guarantee that learners actually *feel* safe.

As part of decolonizing classrooms, we have to be critically conscious of the needs of racialized students and those from minoritized groups who often have experienced microaggressions from other students and professors within educational spaces (Battiste, 2013; Lewis et al., 2019; Matias, 2013). Hence, how do we ensure the brave space has been prepared and ready for risk-taking that involves sharing and retelling of trauma? Cultivating brave spaces begins with not making assumptions and suspending judgement from a stereotypical deficit lens. Some learners rely on forgetting as a survival mechanism to avoid being retriggered when talking about emotionally charged topics. In some instances, this coping mechanism helps students maintain just enough emotional energy to complete the course and engage in the academic rigour required to succeed. Others may rely on silence as a form of resistance and subversion (Eizadirad & Portelli, 2018) to constructively spend their energy.

In contrasting safe and brave spaces as concepts throughout this chapter, we explore "How do you cultivate brave spaces to take risks to challenge oppression?" Creating spaces that are open to sharing pain and trauma is risky and dangerous work, as expression of emotions can be interpreted as a weakness (Eizadirad & Campbell, 2021; Hanna, 2019; hooks, 2002; Matias, 2013). This is part of the normalized neoliberal model of education that promotes neutrality over expression of emotions and feelings labelling strong emotional expressions as unsuitable or unprofessional (Giroux, 2003; Portelli & Konecny, 2013; Rodriguez, 2019; Weiner, 2014). This needs to be disrupted through counternarratives of pain and suffering as critical pedagogy. The term *cultivate* emphasizes intentionality in how we do things and for what purposes, as brave spaces do not just happen by accident. Social justice conversations about topics such as white privilege, anti-Black racism, anti-Indigenous racism, homophobia, and anti-Muslim racism, amongst others, by their very nature trigger emotional responses, and if the space is not prepared to take up varying viewpoints in a constructive manner, it can enact harm on students. As Hanna (2019) explains with respect to discussing whiteness in social justice education,

> Being anti-racist does not mean being anti-white. However it does resist promoting whiteness as an ideology. Whiteness is an ideology of domination that is reinforced by what is both spoken and unspoken. This means requiring reflexivity from everyone, even white allies, to monitor the "space" they take in the classroom. It not only necessitates self-regulating the amount of minutes one speaks in class; it also demands maintaining an awareness of one's body language and energy as these relate to others.
>
> (p. 238)

Therefore, it is important from the start of classes to foster an environment that encourages risk-taking and listening to multiple perspectives to better understand activism, power, privilege, and systemic oppression in various contexts. This also includes being conscious of how we engage in conversations from the words we use and tone of voice to being aware of our body language, gestures, and the amount and type of space we take up. This is part of what we model as racialized professors to our students: not to simply survive, but to be brave and take risks by being vulnerable, disrupt with intentionality, and thrive by making the learning space more insightful for everyone by sharing pain and trauma rooted in lived experiences. As Eizadirad and Campbell (2021) emphasize, "As part of disrupting the sanitization and camouflaging of oppression, we share our lived experiences as counter-stories and discuss how it is a mobilizing force in reinforcing activist pedagogies, facilitate healing from traumatic experiences, and disrupt and promote equitable outcomes" (p. 6). This journey is not linear and involves navigating tensions, complexities, and nuances, which through brave spaces can be harnessed as a mobilizing force for taking action against social injustices. Therefore, we must not dismiss emotions or choose to stay in our comfort zones, but rather take calculated risks beyond our comfort bubbles where we indulge and embrace in our emotions as a source of nourishment for leading us in new directions.

Methods and Methodology: Duoethnography Dancing with Critical Race Theory

Reflecting our lived and professional experiences as racialized professors, we utilize duoethnography (Breault, 2016; Lyle, 2018) as a storytelling methodology to share our pain, suffering, and trauma, but to also celebrate our joy, happiness, and resiliency. This trajectory of embracing both positive and negative emotions reflects our growth as educators in shifting our stance and pedagogies from promoting safe to brave spaces. As Breault (2016) points out, duoethnography is polyvocal and dialogical where "the stories of each participant rest in juxtaposition to the other" (p. 2) and this is "deliberate as an attempt to disrupt the type of metanarrative that can emerge from solitary writing" (p. 3). In writing together, our friendship as authors has grown tremendously beyond academics, and we have become more comfortable sharing our authentic selves including our anger, sadness, and disappointment, and past wounds and traumas that impact us to this day.

Lyle (2018) outlines four benefits to the use of storytelling as a transformational method for new possibilities via autobiographical writing: overcoming fear, articulating our realities, mobilizing for change, and revealing possibilities to ourselves (p. 262). We strengthened our storytelling by sharing it with each other as duoethnography and challenging each other's ideas, experiences, and interpretations of such experiences from multiple vantage points particularly CRT. Lopez (2003) outlines a key characteristic of CRT as

> the privileging of stories and counterstories particularly the stories that are told by people of color. CRT scholars believe there are two differing accounts of reality: the dominant reality that "looks ordinary and natural" to most individuals, and a racial reality that has been filtered out, suppressed, and censored.
>
> (p. 84)

We situated our conversations from a CRT paradigm to disrupt deficit-thinking metanarratives about racialized identities and amplify our experiences as racialized professors. Therefore, the content of this chapter, including its methodological approach, was selected with intentionality as part of a counternarrative that engages pain and suffering as a form of strength rooted in critical pedagogy (Leonardo, 2013; Knoester & Au, 2017; Dixson

& Rousseau, 2005; Lopez, 2003). This includes reflecting on how we met as co-authors, the way we developed our friendship over time built on trust and reciprocity, and how we grew together through sharing our vulnerabilities guided by a passion for change and social justice activism in our roles as professors in the field of teacher education. We became each other's support network as the friendship grew, pushing each other to overcome challenges and cope with pain and suffering more constructively. This is not a linear process, as it involves sharing built-up tension with another within a brave framework that fosters truth-telling.

The intersection of duoethnography as a method and CRT as a paradigm provides a framework that not only acknowledges racialized lived experiences as valuable knowledge, but centres expression of racialized pain and trauma as a counternarrative to neutral colour-blindness promoted within educational spaces under the guise of neoliberalism (Hanna, 2019; Matias, 2016; Tuck & Yang, 2012; Yancy, 2016). Within this framework, there are multiple versions and interpretations to any given event, which leads to different emotional responses. Leonardo (2013) adds to this by outlining the interconnection between objective reality and subjective experiences of reality for racialized identities: "Objective reality carries different meanings for racialized subjects, depending on their social location without determining those meanings. Thus, research on race is a good venue to observe the dialectical process between objective constraints and the formation of racialized subjectivity" (p. 600). This is particularly significant in higher education where "discourse centred on neutrality, objectivity, colour-blindness and merit" (Dixson & Rousseau, 2005, p. 22) dominate conversations about social justice, in the process muting or seeking to silence expression of emotions and feelings by racialized identities.

Brave spaces "insists on historical and contextual analyses. And it values the voices of people of colour" (Dixson & Rousseau, 2005, p. 22). As racialized professors, we use storytelling guided by tenants of CRT and duoethnography to centre our histories, who we are, and our struggles and growing pains to disrupt the practice of dismissing emotions and feelings as invaluable in teaching and learning. In line with Indigenous worldviews, the spiritual aspect of teaching and learning has to be centred to cultivate brave spaces. This holistic approach opens new alternative ways to live, grow, and flourish in academia. This approach is process oriented more so than outcome oriented.

In the upcoming sections of this chapter, we share our experiences via back and forth conversations as polyvocal duoethnography. We have found immense value in sharing our stories of pain with each other as well as with our students as a form of advocacy and activism. The process itself is also therapeutic and allows us to build deep connections with others. By embracing and sharing our vulnerabilities, when we feel ready to do so, we have healed in different ways and experienced growth and belonging as we pull strength from each other. This helps us emotionally to continue to advocate and take calculated risks as a form of advocacy to advance equitable outcomes, particularly for racialized faculty, who, as the research indicates, often feel lonely, excluded, and misunderstood (Ahmed, 2007; Eizadirad & Campbell, 2021; Henry & Tator, 2012; Lewis et al., 2019; Mohamed & Beagan, 2019; Yancy, 2016). By sharing our pain, suffering and trauma, on our own terms and at our own pace, we challenge systemic oppression in educational contexts by disrupting the normalizing gaze and its power dynamics that pressure you to conform or risk facing consequences (Weiner, 2014; Kumashiro, 2004; Yancy, 2016). This is where being conscious of power dynamics and one's positionality is critical. This reflects what Madison (2012) outlines as an activism stance explained as the "stance in which the ethnographer takes a clear position in intervening on hegemonic practices and serves as an advocate in exposing the material effects of marginalized locations while offering alternatives" (p. 7).

Risk-Taking in Brave Spaces

Brave spaces are communities where there is an investment in relationship building and development of trust. It is made clear from the start that multiplicity of opinions and experiences is beneficial to all learners to explore the complexities and nuances in social justice issues. This translates into exploring what it means to be complicit, and how and when to call-out and call-in people as part of teaching and learning as a community of learners. Yet, this has to occur with a space that is kind, loving, and supportive yet prioritizes truth-telling even if it makes people uncomfortable.

In recent years various scholars have theorized brave spaces as a concept and what processes it entails in different contexts working with various social groups: Arao and Clemens (2013) write about brave spaces as a new way to frame dialogue around diversity and social justice, Cook-Sather (2016) discusses brave spaces and student–faculty pedagogical partnerships, Herrmann (2017) explores braves spaces in the context of LGBTQ+ at a writing centre in a post-secondary institution, and Gilmour (2021) examines fostering brave spaces around race. Overall, as a theme the literature emphasizes that brave spaces centre and amplify the emotional and spiritual components to teaching and learning and the associated risk-taking in sharing vulnerabilities. Instead of dismissing emotions and feelings, brave spaces work towards harnessing energy from it to mobilize for personal and systemic change (hooks; 2003; Lorde, 1984). In other words, brave spaces do not avoid tension by remaining in comfort bubbles. Instead, brave spaces push learners outside of their comfort zones by engaging with multiple perspectives and experiences to imagine new possibilities and grow in new ways. This leads into calculated risk-taking where norms and hegemonic structures are questioned as part of unlearning to gain a better understanding of the interconnection between power, privilege, and profit in perpetuating inequities and social injustice (Arao & Clemens, 2013; Campbell &

Watson, 2021; Cook-Sather, 2016; Eizadirad & Portelli, 2018; Gilmour, 2021; Hanna, 2019, Herrmann, 2017; Kumashiro, 2000). As Hanna (2019) puts it, "discomfort should be encouraged because in order to dismantle invisible hierarchies of privilege, we must acknowledge their existence" (p. 233).

Ardavan: For a long time I used the term *safe space* in my teachings because I did not know any better. As I delved further into the literature on equity, anti-racism, and decolonization, and engaged in further conversations with racialized colleagues and students, I became more aware of the root causes of systemic issues and how the neoliberal model of education often places blame of outcomes on individuals through deficit thinking instead of examining inequality of access to opportunities. This provided me with the language and the critical literacy to shift towards using the term *brave spaces*, recognizing that there is no space that is 100% safe for everyone. I recognized that there are things I can do as an educator to prepare the space to be more inclusive and foster supportive sharing. For instance, as part of the start of all my classes, I spend a good amount of time getting students to share a bit about themselves to the extent they feel comfortable, discuss differences between equality and equity, and how we can all contribute to creating a brave space, including myself as the professor. This encourages them to reflect on how much space they take up and in what ways. I use gentle reminders to bring people back to this concept as the weeks go on as part of class.

Andrew: Telling and sharing stories of pain and suffering is often interpreted as a weakness by those in positions of power. They assume that the intention of telling these stories is to gain sympathy or make people feel sorry for you. This is another narrative that needs to be disrupted within academic spaces. Many of us who are able to tell our stories, and do so passionately and with intentionality, share them from a place of vulnerability. However, that vulnerability should not be categorized as weakness. Instead, it should be seen as coming from a place of bravery, as it signals our strength, resilience, resistance, and disruptive nature of standing within unsafe and unwelcomed spaces and telling our truth. The term *brave* recognizes we work within educational settings where enacting danger and harm is possible. The risks are not removed, but we are challenged and in that space we invite allies, advocates, and activists as a collective to do the work to ensure safer spaces are indeed created. This is what I model in all my roles in higher education as an administrator and a professor, from how I carry myself centring my Jamaican accent to how I dress and interact with colleagues.

Arao and Clemens (2013) outline five guidelines for facilitating brave spaces. They are agreeing to disagree, not taking things personally, challenging by choice, respect, and no attacks (pp. 143–149). While we agree with all the aforementioned guidelines, we add that it is important to recognize the needs of learners, particularly racialized and minoritized students from an equitable lens to facilitate cultivating brave spaces. This means being approachable as professors and letting racialized and minoritized students know that we see them, appreciate them for arriving to our class being who they are, and reminding them that they belong in academic spaces and not to doubt it. This means avoiding standardized approaches to dealing with challenges that arise, and doing what is best to meet the varying needs of students with respect to context. There is no one-size-fits-all approach to supporting students. In some cases, support for students translates into advocating on their behalf against inequitable university policies that operate under equality paradigms. As racialized professors, we should not only talk about social injustice, but also model how we can tackle it together as a community of learners and from different positionalities and walks of life.

Andrew: In telling our stories there is often an expectation that we tell it a certain way. The expectation especially in spaces when we choose to talk about racism, anti-Black racism, and issues of oppression is that we display and parade our pain. There are absolutely benefits for being brave within such spaces and telling our stories. However, I have also come to realize that there is an expectation to re-live pain and trauma under the white gaze. I have stepped away from that in many of my presentations and lectures. My stepping away from "serving Black trauma" is deliberate. That silence is intentional. When I am intentional about that silence in my moment of telling, it informs the audience that something is missing, and it is an invitation to them to engage in their own unlearning and to be intentional about what they do with my story, what they do with their emotions, what they do with their empathy. It also signals a warning to white identities to think about how they listen to and engage with stories of trauma and pain shared by others.

Ardavan: In classes where students get marks for professional engagement and participation in class, I emphasize the importance of recognizing and reading power dynamics in a learning environment and encourage learners to come out of their comfort zones to contribute to growing the space beyond personal gains. This means that some students need to participate less as they tend to dominate conversations, whereas others need to push themselves to speak up more. Regardless of the varying needs of the learners, I make sure they know I am there to facilitate respect, truth-telling, and love, and to model it through my words and actions. This also means helping students be conscious of their body language and gestures and how this is an important aspect of engaging in constructive dialogue and discussions. It is not just what you say, but how you say it. I also provide different mediums for people to participate and express their ideas, opinions, emotions, and experiences, recognizing not everyone wants to share their pain and trauma in a large setting where they may not have established trust with others. For example, I offer the option of sharing via online discussion boards or via personal reflections submitted directly to me for students to express their emotions and feelings. This flexibility and differentiated instruction provides multiple entry points for students to engage with the course content and make connections to their own lives and lived realities. These are baby steps towards switching to a growth mindset as a community of learners rather than being fixated with grades and marking. In some of my classes, I have begun to implement ungrading where students only receive feedback for improvement instead of getting letter grades. This is part of challenging systemic oppression in schools and colonial policies that seek to regulate how learning should take place and in what ways over a predetermined length of time, such as a term or semester. This neoliberal logic guided by capitalism has made education all about the type of jobs you can get, which as a system at all levels has marginalized the spirit, soul, and passion of so many learners due to a curriculum that is not socioculturally relevant or sustaining in its content or pedagogies.

Andrew: In my workshops and classes, I find that so many participants arrive with the notion that if we identify places and spaces within our institutions as safe, then it would turn out to be safe just because we say so. The concept of providing a safe space without any real support or intentional strategies to cultivate relationships and trust amongst learners has led to a false sense of safety for many vulnerable persons. I am very happy to see that more and more of those impacted within our institutions are speaking up about the creation of safe spaces that are superficial, performative, and oftentimes more dangerous than productive. We do not begin as a safe space. We begin at a brave space. As marginalized people, resistance and revolt have always been part of our existence. The creation of any brave space begins with both the users and allies being brave and working to find common ground in challenging inequities and social injustice. This bravery begins with being honest about the dangers we are seeking safety from. I have seen many dominant and powerful individuals willing to name the dangers within our institutions faced by Black, Indigenous, and other equity-deserving groups by speaking on behalf of such marginalized groups, but refusing to articulate being safe from who or for what. When we are brave enough to call out those forces within our spaces that are dangerous to the growth, development and well-being of our racialized, excluded, and disenfranchised members, then we have truly begun to create a safer space that fosters belonging for all. This begins with bravery – that willingness to engage in the work that is needed to create change knowing there are risks and potential consequences. Brave spaces symbolize the willingness to say that danger lurks within our institutions and we are committed to eradicating it.

Ardavan: I am big on theory being enacted via actions which reflect the saying "actions speak louder than words." I spend quite a bit of time early on in my classes getting students to express what pronoun they self-identify with, how to pronounce their names, and what name or nickname they prefer to be called by. These are all strategies to foster belonging within the space and building rapport with students. This also contributes to setting the tone for equity conversations to take place in a manner that respects different lived experiences. Many students have shared with me that there are so many times that professors talk about equity as part of course content, but when it comes to supporting them, they operate from an equality paradigm that reinforces a one-size-fits-all approach to different needs and circumstances. Many students face microaggressions from their professors when asking for additional support such as assignment extensions or adaptations to meet their needs. They have shared with me that in many cases professors mention how their hands are tied by university policies where students are told to conform and follow the rules or face consequences. At what point do we, as professors, stand by our students, and as a collective and in solidarity challenge inequitable educational policies and practices? How can we be strategic together to challenge systemic oppression? By the end of my courses, through group activities and collective discussions about social justice issues and what can be done about them in the short and long term, I strive to make students understand that at the heart of research, teaching, and learning is advocacy and activism to learn, unlearn, and grow to challenge systemic inequities. This goes beyond worrying about what job you can get upon graduation.

Disrupting and Breaking the Psychological Shackles of the Baby Elephant Syndrome

The healing and transformative processes that occur within brave spaces allow for breaking free from the baby elephant syndrome and working in solidarity with others towards personal and systemic change. When baby elephants are being trained at a young age, they are chained to a structure to break them psychologically into accepting submissiveness. In order to break the baby elephant to accept subordination, physical and psychological tactics of harming are used to reinforce domination. The baby elephant, who is not as strong as a grown elephant, resists to the best of its ability by trying over and over to break free to the point of exhaustion. It eventually accepts defeat and subordination in its psyche and stops resisting. For the rest of its lifetime, the elephant believes that it is not strong enough to break free from the chains based on its experience as a baby elephant. This belief remains so strong that it prevents them from taking risks again and venturing to try again. This state of accepting defeat is referred to as the *baby elephant syndrome*, where one allows prior negative experience to perpetuate doubt in the psyche and as a consequence disengage from similar opportunities in the future. This is why when elephants are paraded at the zoo, often chains or ropes are placed on their ankles which symbolize learned helplessness in the psyche of the elephant.

Many racialized and minoritized students and faculty suffer from baby elephant syndrome as a result of prior negative experiences. For example, in educational spaces, such as teacher training programmes, discussions are used as a common teaching strategy to explore multiple perspectives on social issues. Many racialized students have shared with us that within such spaces the weight and burden of sharing is thrusted upon them as racialized identities; being seen as the spokesperson about Black or Muslim issues (Matias, 2016; hooks, 2003; Yancy, 2016). The power dynamics in the classroom compels them to share their pain and trauma due to discussions gravitating away from their experiences and not addressing the systemic root causes of their pain and suffering. Therefore, they choose to speak up with intentionality to help others gain a greater understanding of the complexities involved and unlearn to challenge systemic oppression. In some cases this unlearning is also needed for the professor who is reinforcing harm by putting pressure on racialized students to speak up about what is being discussed. Students who share their pain and trauma within spaces that are not supportive nor organized to foster support and healing experience retraumatization with the potential to disengage from the class. This can be attributed to not feeling safe or supported enough to be brave about their personal wounds and vulnerabilities. As Verduzco-Baker (2018) points out, "If marginalized students are the only source of personal experiences of oppression, they are put in a bind: they must either disclose painful experiences or allow denigrating comments to stand. In either case, these students carry an excess burden" (p. 588).

Disrupting and breaking the psychological shackles of baby elephant syndrome is at the core of cultivating brave spaces that facilitate unlearning and overcoming traumatic experiences. Many of us, particularly racialized and minoritized identities, suffer from baby elephant syndrome having allowed one or multiple negative experiences to dictate how we view our own strengths, competencies, and potential. We have internalized oppression based on colonial ideologies and exposure to constant stereotypical representations about who we are, our histories, and what we can achieve (Ahmed, 2007; hooks, 2002; Karumanchery, 2005; Kumashiro, 2004; Leonardo, 2013). This has systemic roots in the discursive discourse around power, privilege, and profit relating to who can produce knowledge and in what ways (Battiste, 2013; Freire, 1970; Giroux, 2003; Leonardo, 2013; Lorde, 1984; Weiner, 2014; Yancy, 2016). For example, how many of us think we are not good at math due to prior negative experiences of doing poorly in a math class or having negative interactions with a math teacher? How many of us are unhappy with how we look or feel unpleasant about a certain body part such as eyes, nose, or skin colour due to what the media socially constructs as ideal beauty affiliated with whiteness and being skinny? These are real-life examples which have implications for how we suffer from baby elephant syndrome rooted in colonial ideologies and logic that socially construct what is normal. What is normalized becomes hegemonic and by essence privileged without it being questioned. Those who deviate from the norm in terms of their attitudes, behaviours, or emotions are often marginalized and oppressed for going against the grain. Cultivating brave spaces is a starting point to break free from the psychological shackles of baby elephant syndrome and to promote calculated risk-taking that facilitates unlearning and healing to take collective action against systemic oppression.

Shifting from Deficit Thinking to Understanding Root Causes of Systemic Oppression

Although one of the guidelines by Arao and Clemens (2013) for cultivating brave spaces is agree to disagree, it is important to go one step further to understand multiple perspectives, particularly the why behind an opinion or perspective that differs from your own frame of reference. This is a critical exercise to deconstruct the complexities and nuances in social (in) justice and deficit thinking ideologies that students come to class with. This is what Freire (1970) called dialogical practice with the goal of creating critical consciousness to inspire personal freedom and challenge systemic oppression. Given normalized power dynamics in higher education, racialized students have unique experiences as part of class discussions about social justice issues compared to non-racialized white students (Lyle, 2018; Matias, 2016). Therefore, "[t]he term 'brave space' then presents entirely different connotations for minority groups of students in contrast to the privileged majority" (Herrmann, 2017, p. 5). As Hanna (2019) emphasizes, "[T]he education of white people cannot depend on the revictimization of people of color" (p. 230). To minimize harm, as educators we must prepare the space for disagreements in a manner that is constructive for healing and growth rather than insulting, unsupported, and oppressive. If this preparation is not done, it can lead to perpetuating further harm for marginalized and racialized students. This level of support is unique for all students given their identities including aspects of race, class, social class, sexuality, religion, and other axes of difference from an intersectional lens. As Weiner (2014) states, "It's forgetting that is made invisible by highly refined techniques of remembering" (p. 59). How often are assignments and assessments predominantly text-based and rely on writing? Whose pain does this privilege and whose pain does it oppress and marginalize with respect to how it can be expressed? What representations and voices do we amplify as part of selecting course content for our classes? What are the positionalities of the authors and are they discussed with the class? Do students have a say in how they can express and demonstrate their learning? Are lived experiences encouraged to be shared? Are they treated as valuable and worthy knowledge? How is theory and practice aligned or are they fragmented?

Ardavan: With intentionality, I have gravitated away from 10- to 15-page papers in many of my courses as the culminating assessment. More recently, I have replaced the lengthy paper with infographics, social media posts with descriptions, and public service announcement video projects that centre activism and advocacy as a key skill to master. This requires students to mobilize and work collaboratively to disrupt metanarratives rooted in deficit thinking by producing counternarratives that raise awareness about social justice issues. Based on the quality of the work and feedback from students on course surveys, I have found these projects more enjoyable both for myself and for the students. These alternative assignments provide a medium to demonstrate higher-level critical thinking. Furthermore, it provides the flexibility for students to apply theory to action based on their interests and passions. In this process, students become advocates and embody activism through their actions and the type of knowledge they produce. This involves discussing strategically where they can make the most impact with the work they do.

Andrew: Growing up in Jamaica I had been accustomed to seeing assessment and evaluation as a time for judgement; a time to weed out; a time to prove who is able, capable, and allowed. Having the opportunity to teach in many other Caribbean spaces, living in the Bahamas, teaching in the USA for a short stint, and finally moving to Toronto, I realize that this notion of assessment as a weapon or weeding out tool is way more widespread. Students will enjoy a course and once it is time for assessment, fear and anxiety step in. I have long questioned this as an educator. I have long questioned why the loss of joy during assessment. This started within my graduate studies in courses where professors were often reluctant to student input in the assessment and evaluation process, where I would present to my professors other possible and interesting products I could use to demonstrate my learning. This was an intentional way to demonstrate that we can move away from the one-size-fits-all practice. This continued when I began teaching in higher education institutions and began to have more insight and questions about the intention of certain assignments. Deliberately, I changed some of those assessments, especially for students who are members of equity-deserving groups to feel brave enough to challenge their own ideas, produce amazing stories and counternarratives, situate and cement their identity through their work, and express and expel pain and trauma constructively. In that process they have produced artefacts that tell their own stories authentically, celebrate their strengths and belonging, and demonstrate the myriad ways in which they will take this very learning into their own classroom spaces. These assessment ideas have empowered Black and other racialized voices, especially in courses deliberately created with the intention to do just that.

To gain a greater understanding of the root causes of systemic oppression one has to learn to listen without interrupting and avoid presenting a simplified right/wrong binary when discussing actions and behaviours of people. Analysis of power has to be central in understanding the why behind behaviours and access to opportunities. This is something that needs to be constantly revisited as we work towards cultivating brave spaces over time. As Gilmour (2021) puts it, "Brave, *sacred truth* spaces must be continuously protected and reenacted throughout the year. It is an active process rather than a destination" (p. 3). This active process needs to be enacted throughout class whenever a difference in opinion arises. Shying away from deconstructing tension in differences can further perpetuate harm and create a toxic environment for students contributing to them feeling invisible, ignored, or excluded. As Cook-Sather explains (2016):

> Brave space, on the other hand, implies that there is indeed likely to be danger or harm – threats that require bravery on the part of those who enter. But those who enter the space have the courage to face the danger and to take risks because they know they will be taken care of – that painful or difficult experiences will be acknowledged and supported, not avoided or eliminated.
>
> (p. 1)

Cultivating brave spaces involves intentionality knowing that conversations about social justice impact people emotionally. Creating brave spaces that are supportive recognizes the needs of the learner relative to their identity and lived experiences and encourages risk-taking. Visibilizing our wounds is for us, led by us. A common practice is the hijacking of our pain and suffering by non-racialized white identities. The hyper-visibility of our pain, packaged and constructed for consumption is problematic as a process. The authenticity of who tells these narratives and how it is told is just as critical as the content of the experience. This brings us back to the notion of gravitating away from the right/wrong binary framework and centring power as the main framework for analysis. Within this framework, we have to work to understand how identities and communities are privileged and oppressed, and how they can mobilize and work in solidarity with allies and others to challenge systemic barriers.

Ardavan: Love/hate, happiness/sadness, and smiling/crying are all complex emotions that are not binaries. There is a range of feelings and emotions in between these binaries. As educators advocating for cultivating brave spaces, it is important to dedicate time, effort, and energy in our classes to deconstruct course content, the positionality of authors we bring into our classes, and the unexpected teachable moments that arise to check in with our students. In the process, we must reciprocate what we ask of our students. I also take risks along the way and share personal matters with my class so the power dynamics of engaging in brave spaces is multilateral and not one-dimensional. This involves sharing with the class what I am passionate about and finding opportunities to collaborate from community work to research. As a result, I have published many papers with graduate students, ensuring they are credited as first authors for doing the majority of the work, and learning skills along the way. In many cases, students are exploited by professors for their labour. As well, I have learned to read the signs that trigger me rooted in my past traumas and growing up in a hyper-masculine environment playing competitive basketball and growing up in a racialized under-resourced community in Scarborough, Ontario. Now when anger comes, I indulge in it, and then learn to let it go, instead of holding on to it. When I let it go, it no longer holds power over me. This has taken tremendous critical consciousness on my end to learn and master. It comes with the maturity of not being fixated on perfection.

Andrew: I always ensure there is a call to action. That call is about connecting their gaze to action. It is a call for others to decide what they do with these stories. How will they be transformative and disruptive to a system that still holds others captive? How do they plan to use their power and privilege to assist in changing those stories of pain and suffering into ones of change and triumph? Stepping away from the ruler of what is prescribed is powerful. For me, it gives me the control of what to share, when to share, and how to share. I have had occasions where the learning community has been created in such a way where I feel compelled to share so much, knowing that there is a level of preparedness and readiness among the learners that this retelling will be effective and therapeutic. In other cases, I have refused to share and retell based on the fact that this particular learning space feels hostile and my reliving of pain and trauma would not be educative or inspirational, but more entertainment and an ungrateful consumption of my story. That is a skill to be developed by many of us as we tell our stories. When do we choose to tell our stories and in what measure? Knowing the power in owning your story gives you this competence and authority. In the powerful lyrics of Lauryn Hill in the song "I Get Out" I am reminded of the urgency in which I must get out of the boxes that have been created for me, boxes I have been forced in based on my complex identities. It is a bold action to get out of boxes that have long been designed and established by historical and systematic oppressive institutions to fit into or face consequences.

> I get out, you can't hold me in these chains
> …
> I won't be compromised no more
> I can't be victimized no more
> I just don't sympathize no more
> 'cause now I understand
> You just want to use me
> You say "love" then abuse me.
>
> (Lauryn Hill, 2002, "I Get Out")

Ardavan: It is transformative and healing to be vulnerable and harness that therapeutic energy to mobilize for personal and systemic change. The processes involved are not perfect. There will be challenges within brave spaces, but those challenges are opportunities to grow in new ways. Sometimes it is a bit of trial and error, but it becomes all about exploring new possibilities through new approaches and perspectives. It becomes about growth and the collective community. We are beyond the labels put on us. Within brave spaces, we are grounded. Within brave spaces, we proudly wear our pain and identities on our sleeves as a form of strength. We seek to be forces unapologetically, spreading advocacy and activism at every opportunity to dismantle a system that is obsessed with reproducing unequal relations of power. We want to be beyond filling in a diversity quota. There is no such thing as a 100% safe space. So the goal is progress and growth to move the needle to safer compared to before.

Andrew: The creation of safer spaces begins within each one of us. Creation for me is an intentional act. It is a deliberate act. It is a choice act. It is about taking action to make changes. Something is created to be of use, to create ease, or to create possibilities. One of those brave creative processes is the work of disrupting from within. Many of us who are engaged in the fight for equity and social justice work within the very same institutions where we are seeking to create these safer spaces. I believe that we often fail in our attempt because we have not counted the personal cost of being a designated disruptor. The idea of disruption within the last two years has gained much attraction. Is it ever safe to push against the structure built within institutions to maintain order and norm? The work of disruption from within speaks totally of a brave stand. It is a conscious acknowledgement that you are seeking to break down barriers that were intentionally designed to be upheld through a normalizing colonial logic affiliated with deficit thinking. It is an acknowledgement that you are seeking to disrupt the usual flow that many institutions have come to deem normal for decades and centuries. Is this ever safe work? I doubt it. Is this brave work? I totally believe it.

Conclusion

Overall, we argue that brave spaces are a counternarrative to the safe space discourse and language that is performative and perpetuated within many educational settings. Brave spaces require working to disrupt with intentionality. Brave spaces encourage calculated risk-taking and foster relationship building and centring emotional and spiritual components of teaching and learning as a community of learners. This requires taking into consideration the unique positionality of learners and their needs and lived experiences. Brave spaces advocate for equity over equality to advance social justice via a pedagogy of engaging with pain and suffering.

Engaging in brave work and by essence risk-taking within brave spaces can be rewarding. It is not a linear trajectory but one that holds potential for new beginnings that can be therapeutic and transformative. We refer to expressions of Black joy and rhythms of Middle Eastern dancing as a symbolism that embodies our radical love and passion to remain true to what we believe in, to rise above the pressures to conform to colonial logics and expectations, and to disrupt with intentionality. We continue to engage in calculated risk-taking despite experiencing negative emotions such as anger, sadness, and disappointment on some days. The joy of doing and being part of equity work, both personally and with others, triumphs the challenges and allows us to bravely step in new directions and challenge the status quo as part of developing meaningful relationships with others and fostering deep connections to our ancestry and lands.

As readers, we invite you to be part of brave spaces holistically including your soul, spirit, and emotions by embracing your vulnerabilities and sharing them with others. This is a form of strength rather than a weakness. Black joy and Middle Eastern dancing as metaphors embody the soul, spirit, and emotions in a beautiful manner that can be interpreted in so many ways; as part of risk-taking to thrive and grow in new ways, to connect with the past, examine complexities of the present, and be intentional in how we approach the future. In brave spaces, we stand on the shoulders of our ancestors and take moments to pause, take a deep breath, and give gratitude as we work towards our inner transformation and strategize as a collective to better our communities. We feel it is our duty to put forth our joy, not as a means of avoiding the pain or the struggle and its implications, or to say we are invisible or not hurt, but expressing that we do not feel hopeless, and that we have a capacity to make a change with hope, faith, and community.

References

Ahmed, S. (2007). A phenomenology of whiteness. *Feminist Theory, 8*(2), 149–168.

Arao, B., & Clemens, K. (2013). From safe spaces to brave spaces: A new way to frame dialogue around diversity and social justice. In Lisa M. Landerman. (Eds.), *The art of effective facilitation: Reflections from social justice educators* (pp. 135–150). Stylus Publishing, LLC.

Battiste, M. (2013). Possibilities of educational transformations. In Marie Battiste (Ed.), *Decolonizing education: Nourishing the learning spirit* (pp. 175–191). UBC Press.

Bourdieu, P. (1999). *The weight of the world: Social suffering in contemporary society.* Stanford University Press.

Breault, R. A. (2016). Emerging issues in duoethnography. *International Journal of Qualitative Studies in Education, 29*(6), 777–794.

Campbell, A., & Watson, K. (2022). Disrupting and dismantling deficit thinking in schools through culturally relevant and responsive pedagogy. In A. Gelinas-Prolux & C. Shields (Eds.), *Leading for systemic educational transformation in Canada: Visions of equity and social justice* (pp. 115–135). University of Toronto Press.

Cook-Sather, A. (2016). Creating brave spaces within and through student-faculty pedagogical partnerships. *Teaching and Learning Together in Higher Education, 18,* 1–4.

Dixson, D. A., & Rousseau, K. C. (2005). And we are still not saved: Critical race theory in education ten years later. *Race, Ethnicity and Education, 8*(1), 7–27. https://doi.org/10.1080/1361332052000340971

Eizadirad, A., & Campbell, A. (2021). Visibilizing our pain and wounds as resistance and activist pedagogy to heal and hope: Reflections of 2 racialized professors. *Diaspora, Indigenous, and Minority Education*, 1–11. https://doi.org/10.1080/15595692.2021.1937600

Eizadirad, A., & Portelli, J. (2018). Subversion in education: Common misunderstandings and myths. *International Journal of Critical Pedagogy*, 9(1), 53–72.

Freire, P. (1970). *Pedagogy of the oppressed*. The Continuum International Publishing Group Inc.

Gilmour, G. I. (2021). Fostering brave spaces for discussions about race. *Middle Grades Review*, 7(1), 1–8.

Giroux, H. (2003). Spectacles of race and pedagogies of denial: Anti-Black racist pedagogy under the reign of neoliberalism. *Communication Education*, 52(3–4), 191–211.

Hanna, K. B. (2019). Pedagogies in the flesh: Building an anti-racist decolonized classroom. *Frontiers: A Journal of Women Studies*, 40(1), 229–244.

Henry, F., & Tator, C. (2012). Interviews with racialized faculty members in Canadian Universities. *Canadian Ethnic Studies*, 44(2), 75–99. https://doi.org/10.1353/ces.2012.0003

Herrmann, J. (2017). Brave/r spaces vs. safe spaces for LGBTQ+ in the writing center: Theory and practice at the University of Kansas. *Peer Review*, 1(2), 1–16.

Hill, L. (2002). I get out [song]. *MTV Unplugged No. 2.0*. Columbia.

hooks, b. (2002). Rock my soul: Black people and self-esteem. In *Beyond Words*. Atria Books.

hooks, b. (2003). *Teaching community: A pedagogy of hope*. Routledge.

Jones, S. M. (n.d.). An invitation to a brave space. Retrieved from https://www.grossmont.edu/faculty-staff/participatory-governance/student-success-and-equity/_resources/assets/pdf/brave-space-poem.pdf

Karumanchery, L. (2005). *Engaging equity: New perspectives on anti-racist education*. Detselig Enterprises Ltd.

Knoester, M., & Au, W. (2017). Standardized testing and school segregation: Like tinder for fire? *Race, Ethnicity and Education*, 20(1), 1–14.

Kumashiro, K. (2000). Toward a theory of anti-oppressive education. *Review of Educational Research*, 70(1), 25–53.

Kumashiro, K. (2004). *Against common sense: Teaching and learning toward social justice*. Routledge.

Leonardo, Z. (2013). The story of schooling: Critical race theory and the educational racial contract. *Discourse: Studies in the Cultural Politics of Education*, 34(4), 599–610.

Lewis, J. A., Mendenhall, R., Ojiemwen, A., Thomas, M., Riopelle, C., Harwood, S. A., & Browne Huntt, M. (2019). Racial microaggressions and sense of belonging at a historically white university. *American Behavioral Scientist*, 65(80), 1049–1071.

Lopez, R. G. (2003). The (racially neutral) politics of education: A critical race theory perspective. *Educational Administration Quarterly*, 39(1), 68–94.

Lorde, A. (1984). *Learning from the 60s. Sister outsider: Essays and speeches*. Ten Speed Press.

Lyle, E. (2018). Possible selves: Restor(y)ing wholeness through autobiographical writing. *Learning Landscapes*, 11(2), 257–269.

Madison, D. (2012). *Critical ethnography: Methods, ethics, and performance*. SAGE Publications, Inc.

Matias, C. E. (2013). Tears worth telling: Urban teaching and the possibilities of racial justice. *Multicultural Perspectives, 15*(4), 187–193.

Matias, C. E. (2016). *Feeling white: Whiteness, emotionality, and education*. Brill Sense.

Mohamed, T., & Beagan, B. L. (2019). 'Strange faces' in the academy: experiences of racialized and indigenous faculty in Canadian universities. *Race, Ethnicity and Education, 22*(3), 338–354. https://doi.org/10.1080/13613324.2018.1511532

Portelli, J., & Konecny, P. C. (2013). Neoliberalism, subversion, and democracy in education. *Encounters on Education, 14*, 87–97.

Rodriguez, C. (2019). Untitled XI. *Scholarship of Teaching and Learning in the South, 3*(2), 102–109.

Tuck, E., & Yang, K. W. (2012). Decolonization is not a metaphor. Decolonization: Indigeneity, *Education and Society, 1*(1), 1–40.

Verduzco-Baker, L. (2018). Modified brave spaces: Calling in brave instructors. *Sociology of Race and Ethnicity, 4*(4), 585–592.

Weiner, E. (2014). *Deschooling the imagination: Critical thought as social practice*. Paradigm Publishers.

Yancy, G. (2016). *Black bodies, white gazes: The continuing significance of race in America*. Rowman & Littlefield.

3 Moving from Oppression to Opportunity

Bringing Light to Educational and Historical Contexts in Critical Pedagogy

Allyson L. Watson, Ameenah Shakir, Sundra D. Kincey, Reginald K. Ellis, and Darius J. Young

Our History: A Recount of Historical Experiences through an Educational Lens

"Tulsa is burning!" yelled residents in the neighbouring village of Rentiesville, Oklahoma. The news spread slowly through the rural town and eventually caught the ear of a young six-year-old boy named John Hope Franklin. His father, Buck Colbert (B.C.) Franklin, had moved to the "big city" just a few months earlier to open a law practice, and Franklin, his mother, and siblings were just days away from reuniting with him in Tulsa before the beginning of the riot. Rentiesville had no telephones or telegraphs and could only depend on the local newspaper, *The Daily Phoenix*, for any information. They learned that many Black people lost their lives, and practically all of Black Tulsa had been destroyed. According to Fain (2017), he recounts that Franklin's mother, Mollie Parker Franklin, a schoolteacher, tried her best to ease her children's fears and assure them that their father was safe. "It seemed like years before we learned a few days later that my father was safe," recalled Franklin. "The significance of the Tulsa riot to me was that it kept our family separated." His mother left for Memphis in December 1921, but Franklin would not leave Rentiesville until four years later. His father survived the riot, but rioters destroyed everything he owned. In the riot's aftermath, B.C. Franklin began practising law under a tent and successfully challenged a city ordinance before the Oklahoma Supreme Court that allowed its Black residents an opportunity to rebuild. Franklin's experience in Tulsa symbolizes the story of many other Black Tulsans during the height of Jim Crow. It is a story of Black excellence, community, and self-determination that built the Greenwood District, also known as "Black Wall Street," during the first two decades of the twentieth century. The community represented a freedom that many Black people, then and now, rarely experienced (Ellsworth, 1992). It is also a story of how Black self-sufficiency and success posed as large of a threat to white

DOI: 10.4324/9781003205296-4

supremacy than any other fictive stories white mobs conjured up to justify their ritualistic, vigilante acts of violence against the Black community.
Finally, the Franklins' story also represents Black resistance and resilience
in the face of white supremacy. B.C. Franklin defiantly erected a tent in the
heart of the Greenwood community, challenged their racist laws, and won
the rights for Black people to begin rebuilding in their community. The
ongoing fight for reparations and retelling of these stories serve as a legacy
of that same spirit of Black resistance.

Unfortunately, the story of Tulsa is the story of hundreds of other Black
self-sufficient communities, which consisted of Black people from all economic classes, that white supremacists have destroyed through overt violent
acts or systemic racism. White perceptions of Black economic and political
power have been routinely countered by the mass murder and destruction
of Black communities through deputized anti-Black racist vigilante violence.
This type of destruction was seen in 1866 in Memphis, Tennessee; again in
1906 in Atlanta, Georgia; and also in 1920 in Ocoee, Florida. As mentioned
earlier, the effects of economic oppression and racism were detrimental to
businesses and individuals in Tulsa, Oklahoma, in 1921. Unfortunately,
more evidence of oppression was documented in history in other areas of
the south, specifically Rosewood, Florida, in 1923; and the eastern states
of North Carolina and Michigan in 1943. While we note these particular
areas, this form of racial violence is not specific to any geographical classification or regional area. It is consistent throughout American history.

The irony of the Jim Crow era is that the system was created to keep
Black people dependent on whites for their everyday survival; however, it
created spaces for Black people to serve their community. As a result, Black
people opened businesses, constructed houses, built schools, participated in
politics, and hosted cultural events without any assistance from their white
neighbours. These communities sheltered their children from the realities of
racism and nurtured a generation of leaders to confront racism after they
left these protective spaces. Neighbourhoods like the Greenwood District
instilled a sense of self-esteem and self-confidence in their children such that
they had very little fear of whites once they encountered them as young
adults. Remembrances of this era of Black economic self-determination,
education, political power, and autonomy should not be overshadowed by
these acts of white terrorism against the Black community. We need to challenge ourselves to move the conversation of Black Tulsans beyond the professional class and speak to the working-class Black people who were killed
and lost everything during the riot.

This chapter answers questions tied to the importance of providing a
counternarrative for educators faced with overcoming the negative claims
that critical race theory should not be taught. Additionally, this chapter calls
for the reader to engage with the past to determine how educators, leaders,
and the like will collectively struggle to move forward to end racial violence
and all other senseless acts of violence in the United States. As such, we

assert that while the disenfranchisement of Black people is actualized, the counternarratives regarding the triumph through the travail and the stories of these experiences shift the lens from the victimized to the lenses of educators, historians, and social justice advocates. The counternarrative written within this chapter illuminates historical occurrences throughout our country from the inception of African American lives stemming from before the Emancipation of the enslaved, through Civil Rights and the Jim Crow Era, *Brown v. Board of Education*, and to and through the Black Lives Matter Movement of today.

1619 and Beyond: How Far Have We Come in the We Shall Overcome Process?

"We Shall Overcome," a gospel song written at the height of the labour strike, became the anthem of strength for African Americans during the Civil Rights Movement. Theology scholar Ralph Jones (1982) illuminated the history of the song, which is best known to represent protest in the midst of a strike from the working class. It derived from a hymn by Charles Albert Tindley in 1901. The song was copywritten in 1976 but has served as a background for Civil Rights films and documentaries for decades. Since before 1619, individuals of the African Diaspora have lived, laboured, and loved on the land that is now the United States of America. Throughout that time, foreigners of this area desired to exert their liberty from an oppressive rule. Thus, in 1776, in Philadelphia, several influential members of early American society decided to draft a document that would bound the 13 colonies not to British rule, but to a new national ideal with its cornerstones of life, liberty, and the pursuit of happiness. In the very midst of these intense dialogues, these founders intentionally accepted "America's Lie" (Glaude, 2020). America's Lie is relative to the notion that if "all people are created equal" there is no struggle for those people based on differences. When in fact, the United States was built on the backs of struggles for Blacks who were torn from their countries. The lie is based on perceived and lauded truth that guises racism, sexual exploitation, brutality, and hatred under a lens of "liberty and justice for all" and the American dream.

As Jefferson, Adams, Franklin, and Madison created and enacted the ideals of what is now the governance for the establishment of the nation, America, there are harsh realities around race and inequity upon its very founding. For example, America was founded as a nation for unity, yet millions of Blacks were legally enslaved. Although the first American to shed blood during the Revolution against the mother country was indeed an African-born man, the founders still embraced the lie that Black folk in America were not human. This lie remains in America's psyche nearly 250 years later. The lie that was created at the very foundation of this nation is the lie that empowered a no-knock warrant to be executed in Louisville, Kentucky, in which Breonna Taylor was shot and killed by the same first-line responders that she worked with. This lie gave George Zimmerman the authority to follow, question, and execute an unarmed Black teenager simply because he decided to walk in the rain. This lie was on full display on May 25, 2020, when Derek Chauvin placed his knee firmly on the neck of George Floyd – despite the pleas of bystanders begging the officer to let Floyd up, and despite the cries of Floyd himself calling out to his mother, who he surely saw as he was transitioning to the realm of the ancestors. Derek Chauvin, George Zimmerman, and the thousands of Americans who have openly lynched Black people have been shielded from prosecution and moral reflection due to America's Lie.

On April 29, 1854, with the founding of the Ashmun Institute (present-day Lincoln University), Black colleges and universities served as what historian Jelani Favors (2019) refers to as communitas of Black political and social development. The Black college movement, unknowingly to benefactors of these early institutions, created a crusade that attacked the concepts of the lie. These institutions developed leaders – religious, educational, and political – who forced America to deal with the lie it created. From Fisk University alum W.E.B. DuBois to John Hope Franklin, scholars informed the world of the history of Africans in America – their civilizations and their culture. The Morehouse Man, Martin Luther King, Jr., forced America to revisit the Declaration of Independence and challenged her to live up to what she said she was on paper. Lincoln University's own Thurgood Marshall, the Civil Rights icon, changed the law to include Black people in all aspects of the judiciary. The aforementioned scholars and activists question how far we have truly overcome oppression in our country. Through new ways and teaching integration, we know that to encourage educators to teach from the lens of acknowledging the historical subjugation and using it as an opportunity to grow as a country, students will develop the cultural and historical insight to progress forward.

Critical Race Theory Overview

During the late nineteenth century, African American scholars grappled with defining the formation of structural racism that laid the foundation for what would become critical race theory. Much of this scholarship centred on the role of education as a primary vector for structural racism, noting the prevalence of segregated schools, lack of state funding, and lack of curriculums that infused African American history in public education, demonstrating the normalization of racial inequity. Notably, African American scholars such as W.E.B. DuBois and Anna Julia Cooper and Carter G. Woodson maintained that the codification of structural racism in Jim Crow educational policies represented a primary form of economic discrimination. As such, a wave of legal challenges to structural racism in education permeated the late nineteenth- and early twentieth-century claims for humanity amongst African American institutions and organizations such as the

National Association for the Advancement of Colored People (NAACP), reaching fever pitch with *Brown vs. Board of Education* in 1954, striking down "separate but equal." To be sure, the *Brown* decision, orchestrated and created by Black legal scholars such as Pauli Murray and Thurgood Marshall at Howard University, provided a route for substantive critiques of the theoretical underpinnings of racial discrimination in the law that produced structural racism. In this regard, legal scholar and activist Derrick Bell (1992, 2000) drew on these broader narratives of structural racism and bias in American institutions, such as education, to produce critical race theory.

In the 1970s, Derrick Bell coined the term *critical race theory*, a legal definition that underscores the historical development and pervasiveness of structural discrimination against Blacks through the codification of laws that reinforce bias. Bell (1992) argued in *Faces from the Bottom of the Well* that America's legal system normalized and bolstered racial exclusion as well as regenerated categories of difference. According to Bell, the normalization of racism in the American legal system reinscribes epistemic violence of Black bodies through policies such as discriminatory hiring practices, for example, quotas restricting access to jobs, culturally insensitive screening of names, unequal pay and promotion, and corporate cultural practices of exclusion for training and management positions. Through mixed-method analysis of violations of Equal Employment Opportunities Commission (EEOC) lawsuits, Bell (1992, 2000) demonstrated American institutions' reliance on categories of difference hindered Black success in legal claims for employment and labour discrimination. Bell (1992, 2000) embedded these ideas into critical race theory as a way to teach law school students about the salience of racial bias in American hiring practices and institutions.

While Bell's (1992, 2000) work significantly changed the trajectory of law school curriculums, it was limited in its discussion of Black women's experiences with employment discrimination. Legal scholar and activist Kimberlé Crenshaw expanded critical race theory by including intersectionality. In 1989, Crenshaw argued that the inextricable linkages between race, gender, and class heightened employment discrimination against Black women (Crenshaw, 2018). Crenshaw's work provided visibility to African American women workers in factories, specifically in the automotive industry. The application of Bell's and Crenshaw's scholarship in legal studies remains essential in programmes with a progressive focus. Unfortunately, both Bell's and Crenshaw's theories have been misquoted, misunderstood, and used as a proxy or catch-all to dismantle diverse learning curriculums in K–12 education. To date, no K–12 school system teaches critical race theory. Yet, according to a 2021 Brookings Institution release, several (eight) state legislative bodies, including Florida, are incorrectly and inappropriately using the phrase "critical race theory" to politicize the resurgence of interest in African American history. The insertion of legislation in an educational theory is concerning to historians and educators. The political misjudgement is based on the thought that critical race theory promotes racism and divisiveness. The authors denounce that misjudgement and assert that critical race theory and the embedding of teaching truths in history allow the learner to understand factual and historical accounts that have happened in the United States and abroad through a critical and inquiry-based lens.

The authors and other proponents of critical race theory and culturally responsive pedagogy believe that the critical conversations help establish a counternarrative of triumph through trial and pose a lens for non-Blacks to understand the pain that was caused and inflicted upon non-whites throughout history. Most critical race theory work focuses attention on accounts of Black history but could also be applied to generations of Jews who suffered during the Holocaust. Furthermore, critical race theory, as a barometer, can offer explanations for the hostility and marginalization of Native American people and tribes that were forcefully and violently moved from their land – the land that was "founded" as America. This paradigm unfortunately, or maybe not, aptly fits the atrocities that took place against Vietnamese people during the Vietnam War, as well as to the truths behind Hiroshima and the Japanese victims of that tragedy. Each of these historical accounts urges the learner, the reader, the student, and the scholar to look closely at how history has shaped itself and how all people involved had very different experiences based on their class, their race, and their place in society. These are difficult accounts to reflect upon, yet, without having conversations about them and delving into the research surrounding them, we miss a historic milestone to learn, grow, and move forward.

Preparing Educators for Difficult Conversations: What Does the Counternarrative Look Like in the Classroom

The transition from historical accounts to present day leads us to look critically at what conversations need to happen across the nation to bring about *racial reconciliation*. Kendi (2016) thoughtfully articulates that with any progress for the Black race, you can often look for regress in historical, educational, and sociological existence.

Since post-slavery and into the Civil Rights era, Black children have had hand-me-down books, less than sufficient classrooms, mediocre supplies, and countless inequities. We follow what has happened after *Brown v. Board of Education* and we still find that almost 70 years after the anniversary, classrooms in the United States still have not changed much for African American students. From Topeka, Kansas, where the ruling for *Brown v. Board* was established, to the Greenwood District of Tulsa, Oklahoma, where the 1921 race massacre occurred, to the hills of Tallahassee, Florida, where injustices in government sparked students at Florida Agricultural and Mechanical University to establish a sit-in for equal rights and service, our people have experienced pain. Through hundreds of years of historical occurrences, there are significant gaps in the opportunity to teach students in K–12 about this pain and establish the stories within history that are taught. There are classrooms in the locations mentioned earlier and those across the country where Black children are still marginalized, hungry, disenfranchised, and live in communities with a digital divide and still cannot access the best education.

In 2014 Watson provided three critical steps for pre-service teachers and early educators to incorporate and to build an inclusive classroom and invite opportunities for historical approaches to pedagogy:

1. School districts can work directly with the historical society, the African American task force, the NAACP, and other educational entities to integrate community and state history for enslaved and oppressed people, and tie the historical happenings to educational teaching standards.
2. Teachers can bring oral history and documented narrative from community figures and historians in the area. School districts can proactively engage community stakeholders in teaching about the pain, trauma, and victory that has come out of it. A similar focus on the Holocaust and the struggle Indigenous people had when they were abused and oppressed should also be shared with learners about African Americans.
3. Infuse cultural and historical accounts within academic literature. Be intentional not just in word but also in deed. Utilize researchers, historians, and educators who are true representatives of the experience rather than people who are unaware and insensitive about culture. Don't engage in false practices if as a district you are not committed to authenticity. Select grade-appropriate curriculum to infuse critical conversations and engaging efforts for teachers, students, and families.

This assertion leads scholars to continue to identify historical ideals in education that have highlighted the lack of clarity, diligence, and intention to shed light on this progress within the education system. Missed opportunities and clouded judgement on the part of teachers who are not willing to discuss what history has done to Black Americans further permeate legislatures and governments pushing agendas to eliminate conversations about race, racial history, racial inequity, and any potential communication about race in the classroom.

What can schools and communities do to incorporate these difficult conversations in a learning context? School leaders and teachers have to be proactive in educating students regarding the historical accounts and the impact on communities. School leaders in districts that were motivated to bring equity and a different perspective to instruction leaned on educational researchers like Geneva Gay and adopted curricular frameworks like culturally relevant instruction. Culturally relevant instruction is a method of integrating student lived and cultural experiences in teaching and educational framework.

Geneva Gay (2010) and Gloria Ladson-Billings (2009) identify key components of culturally responsive educational settings. The literature denotes that culturally responsive teachers have an intentional focus on students' learning needs and that intentionality also includes and maintains a cultural consciousness. Gay further asserts that teachers in a culturally responsive setting work to engage students in a diverse curriculum with a breadth and depth of knowledge of the students' culture within the classroom. Ladson-Billings developed this theory of culturally relevant instruction. It has been widely helpful for schools and communities to work within the confines of the academic curriculum and shape the pedagogical approach to learning by interweaving student culture through acknowledgement and respect. Culturally relevant instruction has been utilized within schools to take specific curricula designed for all students and illuminate teaching methods to benefit students through a cultural lens.

Critical race theory is different, in that it looks at the history of the United States and historical context and provides a counternarrative to misinformation by shedding light on truth and reality for marginalized people. While both are helpful in moving educational spaces through equity, one (culturally relevant instruction) looks at changing curriculum to meet the educational needs of marginalized students, while the other (critical race theory) provides opportunity and the ability to look critically at history and account for the viewpoints of all involved, specifically the marginalized. Added to the discussion is incorporating cultural proficiency and competence across the curriculum so that students receive the information from educators, teachers, and schools that believe and entrust equitable practice. None of the theories or practices bring harm or pose a threat to educational systems; however, the opposers of cultural awareness, pedagogy, and critical race theory believe that by teaching anything outside of the historical norm, there is a possibility of divisiveness in the learning environment and process. Watson (2014, 2017) asserts this truth regarding cultural proficiency in the classroom:

> It is necessary to understand cultural proficiency when considering culturally diverse practice. Cultural competence is the ability to function within or for culture or cultural practice effectively to meet the needs of those in the workplace and social environment. In doing so the culturally diverse practices are delivered with regard to equity and respect for cultural beliefs, behaviors and practices. Working toward cultural competence into cultural proficiency, the latter, provides an organization with behaviors that are not only identified and implemented in practice, but also lead to positive experiences for the diverse population involved.
>
> (Watson, 2014, p. 328)

The ideals that shape what history has taken place in the United States are still relevant to what is happening today around racial disparity and inequity; however, many times, educators have digressed from intentional approaches to catch-all ideas about oppressed cultures. Instead of putting all theories and notions into a catch-all response to equity, educators should be more explicit in ways to increase cultural awareness and include opportunities for learning.

Developing Critical Pedagogy through Intentional Commitment to the Counternarrative

Black Americans have used the art of storytelling for centuries. Through storytelling, history is shared among generations, lifelong lessons are developed, and expressions ranging from joy to anger are displayed (Wilson, 2002). Told by and from the African American perspective, these stories provide a profound truth of eras filled with positive and negative experiences that document the experiences of African Americans within and outside the United States. While these experiences shape the narrative from the narrator's perspective, the perspective begins to shift after being told by others. As stated earlier, the shift in this narrative can be seen well before the emancipation of the enslaved to beyond the Civil Rights era and even today in the wake of tragic events of African Americans declaring their lives matter through the Black Lives Matter Movement.

Chimamanda Ngozi Adichie (2009) iterates the importance of a diversity of stories, voices, and perspectives in her infamous TED Talk "The Danger of a Single Story." According to Adichie, "stories matter." They are essential, she said, to reduce stereotypes of people and places. As breeding grounds for history, personal truths, and intellectual ideologies, the authors of this chapter surmise that educational institutions, K–12 and higher education, have a responsibility to not only represent the narrative as once told but also commit to a counternarrative to preserve the elements of positivity and human dignity. To maintain the stories of triumph and positive commitment of the African American community, there must be a severe and intentional commitment to the counternarrative to tell the story for the next generation. Because educators carry great responsibility for moulding individuals and preparing them for the workforce, they also have a responsibility to enact change. In this context, that enactment of change uses one's voice purposely to ensure that students are provided with the whole truth and not just one's perspective or that shaped by society but filled with gaps.

Earlier, we referenced critical points in history that have become a focal point for Black Americans such as the Tulsa massacre, the Ocoee (Florida) massacre, and racial injustice and harm. Essential in this discussion is the Greenwood District in Tulsa, Oklahoma, a thriving community famously known as "Black Wall Street" in the early 1900s (Clark, 2019). This community is crucial because it was once a prosperous Black community and an essential part of the Black/African American narrative. It should be noted that the development of this community was intentional. It was built in response to Blacks being isolated by white-only businesses (Fain, 2017). The community served its residents with essential companies with Black entrepreneurs, such as newspapers, grocery stores, restaurants, and medical offices. In this context, we mention Black Wall Street because the narrative surrounding this particular community changed drastically following the Tulsa Race Massacre in May of 1921. These riots caused a wave of destruction and essentially destroyed this vibrant community. In addition to businesses being destroyed, historians reported that 300 people died and at least 800 were injured (Fain, 2017). Now 100 years later, in the year 2021, we look back on how the Tulsa Race Massacre changed the narrative of Blacks in America. It is estimated in today's dollars that rioters ruined over $200 million of Black property (Messer et al., 2018). Before the riots of Tulsa, the Greenwood District was an affluent African American community built by its residents. Within just a matter of one to two days, the whole world changed for this community. Its economic power and generational wealth were eradicated.

Incidents such as the Tulsa Race Massacre and the eradication of Black Wall Street provide even more impetus towards a conviction to remain committed to the counternarrative. As once told, Blacks lived and thrived in their affluent community built by and for them. However, with many of the events that have occurred throughout history and today, it is difficult to remember a time when Blacks collectively were a thriving race. As such, it is imperative that institutions of K–12 and higher learning commit to a counternarrative to dispel what many believe to be the truth about specific groups of people, cultures, and ethnic groups, particularly African Americans and Blacks. While we must protect educational autonomy, as educators we must realize that the tragic events of today will become history for future educators and students. Therefore, it is our responsibility to ensure that the narrative today is told in the classroom based on the facts so that future educators may focus on the learning outcomes of students rather than creating a counternarrative to dispel untruths.

For today's students, it is important that we create a space for open dialogue for both K–12 and post-secondary students. Sundra D. Kincey, one of the co-authors of this chapter, notes that creating this safe space for students helps to enrich classroom discussions. In her classes, she encourages dialogue and creates opportunities for mock debates on historical and current events. Her only ground rule is that while students are encouraged to share their true feelings on a topic, their dialogue must be embedded with facts and all commentary of opposing opinions must be done so respectfully. These open discussions allow students to express and acknowledge the pain of their peers. Her hope is that the healthy debates will not only inspire critical thinking but might also provide a healing environment for students who may have internalized the pain and anguish felt by families of individuals who have suffered at the hands of others solely based on the colour of their skin, which is a born identity and not a choice. An African proverb states:

"The true tale of the lion hunt will never be told as long as the hunter tells the story." As educators, we become the voice of reason and truth to tell the story for all to hear without bias and subjectivity, but in its truth to uplift all members of the human race.

Moving from Pain to Progress

Due to the calls for humanity and justice after the terroristic state-sponsored violence and murders of Ahmaud Arbery, Breonna Taylor, and George Floyd during the summer of 2020, many state governments passed voter suppression laws as well as efforts to erase African American history from the K–12 curriculum. During a catastrophic global pandemic, state-sponsored violence protests and calls for diversity and inclusion in academic spaces have been incorrectly deemed critical race theory. Legislators have pushed into educational autonomy and have moved to ban critical race theory and accurate history linked to African Americans to diminish and wipe out the essential perspectives of oppressed people. It should be noted that the chapter authors are two generations removed from the travesties outlined. in this chapter. Even so, the pain our ancestors experienced and endured is carried with us in our daily lives.

While the pain can be overwhelming, we stand on the shoulders of our ancestors and truly are their wildest dream. To have overcome obstacles, to have been provided with no generational wealth, and to have pressed past the negative narrative to create a counternarrative and shape our future generations give us strength to continue. Chapter co-author Allyson L. Watson, as a first-generation college graduate, did not face as many obstacles based on racial inequity as a child or student. It wasn't until her professional career as a teacher began that racial inequity became very real to her. Watson was hired as a teacher in the heart of a Ku Klux Klan (KKK) area in northwest Tulsa, Oklahoma. The school was predominately white with a burgeoning Latino and Black student population. She was hired as one of three Black teachers in the school to meet the need for district diversity. Watson, in her first year of teaching, stood face to face with a leader of the KKK who wanted to remove his child from her classroom because Watson was Black. The economic and racial segregation was prevalent in the Tulsa community and the sting of the Tulsa Race Massacre permeated the northern and southern communities. Schools, neighbourhoods, and churches were segregated throughout Tulsa. Watson used her career experiences as a catalyst to promote unity. She eventually left the K–12 school setting to pursue an education research career. She was eventually hired as an academic faculty and founded a programme to prepare teachers to effectively work in high-need schools. Her research led her to become the first endowed professor at a predominately white institution. Her work and research aligned with a notion of reconciliation and teaching cultural competency in educational spaces.

Kincey, as a first-generation college student, had to overcome many of the obstacles noted in the literature for this group of students, including participating in a sit-in during her early college years, which was well past the Civil Rights Movement. Through perseverance, she succeeded and uses that same dedication and passion to mentor students to find their own self-truths and create a narrative for which they can be proud. Chapter co-authors Ameenah Shakir, Reginald K. Ellis, and Darius J. Young are academic historians and have utilized their higher education career platform to promote truth-telling in history. They have worked in academia, sit on state and national history boards, and co-author other published works about the painful experiences of Blacks in Florida. The positionality of the authors and their lived experiences as a collective helps further the conversation to provide meaningful dialogue and discourse about weighty topics that impact future progress. Together the five authors bring their collective experiences and add to the counternarrative, while providing a nudge for proactive teaching and not reactive explanation.

Conclusion

The current political climate in America is as divided in 2021 as it was a century ago. The long narrative of racial violence and America's desire to ignore this past have produced an education system that has not adequately addressed the race question in America. The authors of the chapter are arguing for a re-examination of curricula and teaching strategies in our public schools. One that presents a counternarrative to the whitewashed, heroic story of American exceptionalism, and instead promotes the development of a multicultural education that embraces the stories and contributions of marginalized groups. Sociologist Charles M. Payne (1984) wrote that it is

> [R]ecognized that there are many who work in today's schools who do not hold a racist attitude. However, unless all educators become aware and knowledgeable of how racism has influenced American education, we run the risk of perpetuating rather than eradicating the effects of racism.
>
> (p. 124)

It has been proven that racism in our schools cannot be cured by policy and legislation alone. Educators must remain committed to amplifying the voices of individuals who have been largely written out of history. Educators must challenge their students, colleagues, and administrators to move beyond false concepts of equal opportunity and instead advocate for an equal chance for Black people. Payne distinguishes between the two by arguing that equal opportunity can be granted by a court decision, but equal chance is probabilistic and depends on nonlegal factors, such as family background. The events used to contextualize the plight of the Black community support this claim. A commitment to telling Black history and embracing the teaching of critical race theory has the potential of increasing achievement in Black students. Educators who move beyond the master narrative of American history and take a multicultural approach to education develop students who are committed to racial equality, and have the skills, proficiency, relationships, and values that are essential to living in a Democratic society. Nelson Mandela once remarked that "education is the most powerful weapon which you can use to change the world." It is the intention of the chapter authors to remain diligent in this pursuit.

References

Adichie, C. N. (2009). The danger of a single story. *TED: Ideas Worth Spreading.* Retrieved from https://www.ted.com/talks/chimamanda_ngozi_adichie_the _danger_of_a_single_story/transcript?language=en

Bell, D. A. (1992). *Faces at the bottom of the well: The permanence of racism.* Basic Books.

Bell, D. A. (2000). *Race, racism and American law.* Apsen Law & Business.

Clark, A. (2019). Tulsa's 'Black Wall Street' flourished as a self-contained hub in early 1900s. Retrieved from https://www.history.com/news/Black-wall-street -tulsa-race-massacre

Crenshaw, K. (2018). Demarginalizing the intersection of race and sex: A Black feminist critique of antidiscrimination doctrine, feminist theory, and antiracist politics. In K. T. Bartlett & R. Kennedy (Eds.), *Feminist legal theory* (pp. 57–80). Routledge.

Ellsworth, S. (1992). *Death in a promised land: The Tulsa Race Riot of 1921.* LSU Press.

Fain, K. (2017, July 5). The devastation of Black Wall Street. *J Daily.* Retrieved from https://daily.jstor.org/the-devastation-of-Black-wall-street/

Favors, J. M. (2019). *Shelter in a time of storm: How Black colleges fostered generations of leadership and activism.* UNC Press Books.

Frierson, M. (2020). *Freedom in laughter: Dick Gregory, Bill Cosby, and the Civil Rights movement.* SUNY Press.

Gay, G. (2010). *Culturally responsive teaching: Theory, research, and practice.* Teachers College Press.

Glaude, E. S. (2020). *Begin again: James Baldwin's America and its urgent lessons for our own.* Crown Books.

Jones, R. H. (1982). *Charles Albert Tindley, prince of preachers.* Abingdon Press.

Kendi, I. X. (2016). *Stamped from the beginning: The definitive history of racist ideas in America.* Hachette UK.

Ladson-Billings, G. (2009). *The dreamkeepers: Successful teachers of African American children.* John Wiley & Sons.

Messer, C. M., Shriver, T. E., & Adams, A. E. (2018). The destruction of Black Wall Street: Tulsa's 1921 riot and the eradication of accumulated wealth. *American Journal of Economics and Sociology, 77*(3–4), 789–819. https://doi.org/10.1111 /ajes.12225

Payne, C. (1984). Multicultural education and racism in American schools. *Theory into Practice, 23*(2), 124–131.

Watson, A. L. (2014). Definitions of culturally diverse practice. In L. Cousins & G. J. Golson (Eds.), *Encyclopedia of human services and diversity* (Vol. 2, pp. 327–328). Sage.

Watson, A. L. (2017). Developing a practice of cultural awareness in pre-service teachers by promoting positive dialogue around diversity. In L. Leavitt, S. Wisdom, & K.Leavitt (Eds.), *Cultural awareness and competency development in higher education* (pp. 223–236). IGI Global.

Wilson, M. L. (2002). African and African American storytelling. *Tar Heel Junior Historian.* Retrieved from https://www.ncmuseumofhistory.org/learning/tar-heel -junior-historian-association/magazine

4 Storying Vulnerability

Creating Conditions for Generative Relationality in International Experiential Service Learning

Jessica Vorstermans

What does it mean to evoke mutuality within and against unequal power relations, between Southern hosts and Northern students in the space of international experiential service learning? Learning about inequity and the lived realities of those in the South, the ways in which global capital marginalizes some bodies, should not be pleasurable; it should be labour-intensive, self-reflexive, difficult and push Northern learners to radical new ways of thinking and being (Andreotti, 2015). This chapter takes up the learning of Northern student participants with a small international experiential service learning (IESL) organization, understanding how participants experienced encounters that are structured to challenge capitalist forms of community (Vrasti, 2012). It focuses on student reflections on vulnerability during their Global South placements with a small international experiential learning programme that worked with Canadian universities and operated on a relational model rooted in a philosophy of "being with, not doing for," and used innovative pedagogical tools to counter the hegemonic charity-steeped benevolent Northerner narratives characteristic of the field of IESL (Heron, 2007; Jefferess, 2012).

University and college students from the North are increasingly being pressed to internationalize their education (Larkin, 2012; Shubert et al., 2009; Tiessen & Epprecht, 2012). Closely linked to the growth in IESL is the desire to build or foster an identity of global citizenship in young people from the North (Huish & Tiessen, 2014). In the field of higher education in Canada, there has been an overwhelming interest in international experiential and service learning opportunities across all disciplines, but there is no agreed upon structure for how this should be undertaken (Huish & Tiessen, 2014). This renders the space diverse and fraught with ethical and moral entanglements, but there is also room for hope and alternatives. I understand IESL as rooted in the colonial legacies, neocolonial and imperial relations of power, and as spaces where students from the North are formed as certain subjects under capital. Throughout this chapter I use the term *we*, implicating myself, in the hierarchies of power and privilege, inequality and ableism, colonialism and imperialism that this study is embedded in. I am a white, cis-gender, currently able-bodied settler researcher and educator

DOI: 10.4324/9781003205296-5

in this space and want to acknowledge that this shapes my work and my relation to this work. I was a participant in the Intercordia programme, the focus of this study, in 2005 and worked with the organization in various capacities, including co-leading the organization near the end of its tenure. I have experience in both the practical implementation of IESL and as an area of study; I am deeply committed to being in this work in complex and generous ways.

Encounters facilitated through IESL programmes often obscure inequity and complexities in order to make the experiences palatable and fun for students from the Global North, and work towards a specific formation of the Northern subject. In these encounters, complexity must be erased, simple stories about helping and fixing are celebrated, and changing the world becomes an easy and indeed fun activity that those from the North are entitled to participate in. David Jefferess (2012) explains the main-stream construction of a global citizen as the Northern subject who "helps an unfortunate Other," retaining the other as an "object of benevolence" (p. 27). Jefferess argues that this climate of benevolent helping obscures privilege and power, the reasons why some live in poverty and others (us) don't. He contends that not everyone can be a global citizen, as it is only certain bodies (Northern) that are deemed able to even engage in this iden-tity formation. Elsewhere, I work through the intersection of disability in this space, highlighting how encounters (re)produce a caring and benevo-lent able-bodied Northern global citizen. I argue that this subject formation relies on two main processes: the creation of an able/disabled binary, where the volunteer is able-bodied and the one being helped is the disabled; and the obscuring of the role the Global North plays in producing impairment (Vorstermans, 2018a).

This work is meant to engage with scholarship in the field of critical IESL, making known the ways that Northern subject making is taking place in this space (Andreotti, 2015; Chouliaraki, 2013; Jefferess, 2012; Heron, 2007; Mahrouse, 2014; Mostafanezhad, 2014; Vrasti, 2012). I take up the invitation to a different encounter with the Southern *other* through a case study of the relational model of Intercordia Canada, rooted in mutuality and vulnerability, asking whether this invites student participants into a space where they can begin to critically analyze and challenge the damag-ing and disabling narratives and pedagogical practices that are present in mainstream IESL. The deep emotional labour of naming and announcing one's own vulnerability challenges the script of the benevolent Northern helper in the field of IESL. In the pedagogy of Intercordia, vulnerability was constructed as a natural part of our interconnected humanness and was employed as a tool to get into the messy and difficult work of creating relationships of mutuality across differences. I take up the ways these tools can reproduce a dangerous equating of vulnerability and pain, and offer-ings of ways that this thinking can be interrupted. I think through the ways a radical engagement with vulnerability can serve as a basis to engage in a relational solidarity with others experiencing poverty and inequity and serve as a generative productive force for change. Intercordia's pedagogical tools, used to elicit students' stories of vulnerability, pain, and suffering rooted in one's own positionality, are meant to offer an invitation to meet others who are living systemic vulnerability and disablement and one's own complicity in complex transnational systems of oppression. I use the term *disablement* as the intersecting processes of (neo)colonialism, (neo)imperialism, and capitalism that create the material conditions and social relations of disability in particular ways for particular bodies; particular inequities that disable certain bodies in specific ways (Gorman, 2016; Grech & Soldatic, 2016).

A critical pedagogy rooted in vulnerability only opens the *possibility* for disruptions of reproductions of disablement and systems of oppression. Radical change requires "long haul work" and there can be no fantasy of "once and for all transformation into allies" of the transnational disability movement and all movements towards justice (Heron, 2007, p. 154). My work operates from this understanding. We need to be patient and faithful in our long haul labour of revolutionary love and systemic change that is relational and inclusive. The narratives I will take up from student participants about their own vulnerability were complex and reflected the desire of the student participants to dig in, to explore what it feels like to stay in one's vulnerability and name it as a time of growth and possibility, and not to make instant moves to cover up or push aside uncomfortable feelings. Participants gave concrete stories of vulnerability; what it looked and felt like to feel vulnerable and where that moved them to in their learning. Their stories revealed how staying in their own vulnerability moved them to deeper and difficult learning, an openness to the *other* as knower and teacher. Last, the pedagogy of vulnerability was also lived through the praxis of mentorship, peer mentors who live with student participants in their overseas placements.

Intercordia Canada's Relational IESL Model

Intercordia Canada was a small IESL not-for-profit organization that partnered with Canadian universities and community organizations in Canada and the Global South and operated from 2003 to 2018. The programme had four major components: a full-year academic course at a partner university; four formation days led by Intercordia staff over the academic year; a three-month international or national placement; and upon return, a two-day reintegration seminar in Canada (Intercordia Canada, 2016). The placements where student participants completed their three-month experiences were in the following countries: Ghana, Rwanda, Honduras, Nicaragua, Dominican Republic, Ecuador, Bosnia and Herzegovina, Ukraine, and nationally in L'Arche communities across Canada. It is necessary to centre that students were supported while in placement in the Global South by a trained Intercordia peer mentor (this was uneven due to the numbers of students to support this model financially). It is this commitment to in-depth and critical preparation, and emotional and reflective support to facilitate deep learning while in placement that characterized Intercordia's commitment to relationality.

The pedagogical invitation to participants was to encounter *others* in the spirit of being *with* and not doing *for* (Intercordia, 2016). It was an invitation to engage in relationships of mutuality with those marginalized as non-normative, but one that did not close the space for the Northern body to transgress non-normative ways of being as well. I engage with this work, but not as an example of a way to counter the irrevocably bad IESL with the inherently good. Instead, I aim to flush out the places where this relational model functions as a different invitation to participants and what narratives on learning come out of this engagement, in all of their complexities. I explore whether Intercordia opened a space where student participants could challenge the organizational forces that shape our consent to our current phase of capitalism and capitalist forms of community, what Vrasti (2012), influenced by Foucault, calls "a more tolerable, equitable, and pleasurable phase/face of capitalism" that "conceal[s] its tensions and postpone[s] its crises" (p. 2).

The invitation from Intercordia to encounter difference, to enter into relationships with those who are different, is not unique in the field of IESL. Indeed the foundational summons of IESL is to meet the *other*, to engage in cross-cultural encounters. The highly specific way Intercordia articulates and scripts this encounter with difference is one based on a call to "being with" and not "doing for" the *other*. The pedagogy challenges the construction of who is imagined as the helper, who is imagined as needing help, and who is entitled to engage in the act of helping. The invitation is to encounter difference by being *with* those who are different, and not by helping or doing for those who are different (Intercordia, 2016). This invitation asks student participants to meet the Southern *other* as expert, knower, and agent of their own lives, society, culture, and country, and not as a passive recipient of helping, saving, or theorizing. Northern students are not invited to help or save; but to meet, to be with, to live with, and to learn from Southern *others*. I was interested in hearing how Intercordia alumni heard this call to encounter difference, how they translated the invitation in their own learning about their encounters with Southern *others*.

The affective experience of IESL can serve as a steam valve for Northern students; the pleasure of giving back to those in the South lulls us into believing that this phase of capitalism is "better" or more benevolent than previous phases (Vrasti, 2010). Encounters are steeped in affective pleasure; the living with Southern hosts in their day-to-day lives and working alongside others in community work is often forwarded as the way Northern students will be transformed into caring, global citizens (Conran, 2011; MacDonald, 2016). The critical literature shows that this affective learning is not a path or prompt to mutuality and solidarity (Mahrouse, 2014; Mostafenezhad,

2014). Instead of sowing seeds for system change, encounters under IESL can become an end in themselves; the feel-good affective experiences that allow Northerners to tolerate the inequities and violence of capital and lull us into an acceptance of the tensions (Vrasti, 2012). Learning about inequity and lived realities of those in the South, the ways in which global Capital marginalizes some bodies, should not be pleasurable; it should be labour-intensive, self-reflexive, difficult, and heartbreaking, and push one to radical new ways of thinking and being, centring one's own complicity in systems of harm.

Methods

This chapter comes from a larger study in which I completed semi-structured interviews with 12 student participant alumni of the Intercordia programme (Vorstermans, 2018b). The interview questions in my study asked Intercordia student alumni to reflect on specific pieces of the three broad tenets of the programme: the value of being with people over doing for them (mutuality), that our own vulnerability allows us to enter into relationship with those around us in deeper ways, and that learning is best done in community (Intercordia, 2016). I asked whether their reflections on their experience in the Intercordia programme create meaningful disruptions to disabling discourses of IESL. I looked for moments of disruption to the disabling discourses that operate on simplistic and binary understandings of complex and structural issues. I identified the times when student participants were open to remaining in complexity, signalling a movement away from the rush to consolation or resolution (Andreotti, 2015, p. 14), which is so natural for Northerners shocked and outraged by what they are learning, yearning for positive and enactable answers that they can engage in.

All of the research participants were student participant alumni of Intercordia and had completed the programme between 2012 and 2014. All were between the ages of 19 and 22 when they completed the programme. They participated in the programme in their second, third, or fourth year of undergraduate study at a number of Canadian universities. Their fields of study were very broad and included political science, social justice and peace studies, psychology, philosophy, global studies, international studies, and anthropology with second majors in Great Books, French, First Nations studies, art history, and thanatology. Three participants had participated in another experiential learning programme before the Intercordia programme, and one had participated in an international volunteer trip not connected to an academic course. Research participants were predominately female, and 25% of the participants were male. They were predominately white, and three research participants identified as Black, Indigenous, or People of Colour (BIPOC). One participant self-identified with a non-normative sexual identity; this came out in a story about difference and acceptance by the Southern *other*. I did not ask whether participants identified as having a disability and no one claimed this identity. Participants spoke openly about their experiences with anxiety and changes in their mental health while abroad in placement, very much following a social model understanding of disability, embedding their experiences in structures outside themselves, and not as a medicalized or individual understanding (Oliver, 1990). I used pseudonyms for all participants and do not mention identifying parts of their stories in order to maintain their anonymity. I am grateful for the importance and care they generously gave to this project.

In this chapter, I aim to illuminate the ways in which the Intercordia invitation and framework is intimately *lived out* by student participants, and the specific ways they talk about how they entered into relationships with Southern *others*. I wanted to know how this framework translated into how they imagined the Southern *other* and how they engaged in the *being with* those who are different. What did vulnerability look like for them, as an individual and in relation to the community they were living in? I work to make known how student participants engaged in mutuality in relationships, and how they imagined this experience for the *other* in the encounter. Are there moments of "mutual valuing of relations and [a] refusal to objectify" (Heron, 2007, p. 68)? The encounters within these experiences are deeply raced, gendered, classed, and disabled. We enter geographical spaces marked by colonial and imperial violence that was and is engaged in by certain bodies upon certain bodies. Student participants are entering into Southern geographical spaces with their Northern bodies, shrouded in privilege and the benevolent helping imperative (Heron, 2007). This of course looks different depending on identity. Razack's (2001) work with racialized social work students in practicum placements is important here. Disruptions to the reproduction of colonial and imperial violence and oppression are possible. It is these moments of interruption I am interested in exploring. In research with host families who welcome Intercordia student participants (MacDonald & Vorstermans, 2015) we found that host families and community members experienced relationships of mutuality with student participants and reported this as a strength of the programme. Hosts told us that they engaged in the programme because it allowed for or made space for encounters of mutuality, a period of time to learn from one another, to share more about each other's world and build relationships.

Storying Vulnerability: Disruptive Stories of Vulnerability in IESL Experiences

Engaging and exploring one's own vulnerability was foundational for Intercordia's invitation to Northern students in their being *with* Southern *others*. In the framing of the Intercordia experience, vulnerability was constructed as a natural part of our humanness; loneliness and isolation are an integral part of the human experience. Vulnerability was employed as a tool to get into the work of mutuality (Intercordia, 2016). This construction was forwarded to enable student participants to stay in a difficult space of learning in a good way. IESL programming often employs the ascribing of vulnerable to the Southern *other* and need for the Northerner to help, rehabilitate, save, and care for that vulnerable *other*. The unruly body is always the Southern disabled body, helped and brought joy to by the Northern helper (Erevelles, 2000). Intercordia intervened in this construction and invited Northern student participants to deeply engage with their own vulnerability, discovering the ways they are vulnerable, and posited that through this self-reflexive process mutuality in relationship with the *other* is possible. The Northerner announcing one's own vulnerability is a way of performing unruliness, disrupting the helper/helpee binary that structures IESL experiences. The deep emotional labour of naming and announcing one's vulnerability challenges the script of the benevolent Northern helper. This labour was supported through active reflection and peer mentorship while Northerners were preparing for their overseas experience and while in placement, in an attempt to have the support of this process not fall to Southern hosts.

I heard a wide diversity of ways in which participants experienced vulnerability in their Global South placements. Participants did not self-identify as helpers, as bearers of knowledge or expertise, and they did not assume they would be capable of navigating the complex social and cultural norms of the host country. Some participants talked about the process of deeply embracing their own vulnerability; the movement from feeling unable to engage, communicate, or be with others to the learning and accepting that this is a natural state, a state of vulnerability that they wanted to stay in and start to learn why this being uncomfortable is a valuable state of being when engaging in encounters across difference. Vulnerability was a sort of freedom for them, a freedom from the scripts of benevolent Northern helper, a script that is a problematically constructed position, an imagined one, and one that cannot be realized, one that is inherently harmful. Intercordia's invitation to acknowledge one's own vulnerability as an integral part of their experience, as the fertile ground for entering into meaningful and mutual relationships allowed them to enter more deeply into encounters with Southern *others*. The permission to acknowledge their own vulnerability, that they are not the saviour of the *other* and that they are not there to help, change, or make better, gave them a sort of freedom from the unattainable, and harmful, position of benevolent helper.

Overall, I heard that student participants felt they were well prepared to live the experience of cultural adjustment, vulnerability, and newness in their overseas placement. However, this preparation did not mean they did not feel overwhelmed and isolated when they arrived. Many expressed that they were surprised at the extent of how deeply they felt this isolation. One student participant, Casey, explained this feeling as "I didn't know how to exist." Student participants talked about knowing, on an intellectual level, that they would feel vulnerable, isolated, and scared, but that the lived experience of these feelings was more overwhelming and difficult than they had anticipated. Each participant who talked through experiencing vulnerability and a sense of isolation and loneliness worked through it as a natural reaction to living in a new culture, and did not externalize this process as being one that was about the environment around them, but instead it was about them being in a new and unfamiliar space. They often named the first one and a half months as very difficult, as a lonely and unsettling time. They did not fully intellectualize what it would be like to live a deep sense of loneliness.

Vulnerability as Difficult and Generative

Living vulnerability was not easy for many participants. There is no dominant cultural script for living vulnerably when one is able-bodied and privileged. The assigning of vulnerability is only for some bodies. One student participant, Casey, talked through the process of embracing their own vulnerability, of how hard it was in the beginning to not know how to *be* in any way that was familiar or known to them. Casey explained that they felt bad that they did not speak the local language, did not know the local sign language, that they felt selfish for imposing on the community, for being there for their own growth and learning, and had anxieties about doing harm. Casey explained that they engaged in internal processing and work in reflecting on why they were feeling these anxieties, and eventually moved to find learning in this state of vulnerability. Casey described it as a movement to being humbled by their experience when they realized that their ascribed worth was a constructed worth:

> I have very few life skills. [Laughter] Well … I am smart, I can, like dance, I can swim. Things, you know you think you can do. That are maybe held here [Canada] as worth something. And then I got there and I was like, no actually I can't cook you guys dinner, I can't clean properly, I don't know how to cut wood, I don't have language skills, I was like – I don't have very many tangible skills. And my host brother, who is like, fifteen, and can do a million things, so it was really humbling, I have so much to learn about life.

Casey was open to challenging what is constructed as valued or meaningful in Northern society, of embracing their new way of being in a culture where they did not have valuable or meaningful skills. Instead of using the South as a space to reify her position as expert or helper (Heron, 2007; Vrasti, 2012), Casey entered into a learning about the construction of what is valued under neoliberalism (social capital) and what are tangible skills (life sustaining and reproducing activities), and the disconnections between the two.

Another student participant, Jamie, worked through the invitation to vulnerability as a tool to challenge their self-described "simplistic" understanding of feminism as one that centres on women taking power. Here vulnerability led to a generative learning, a deepening in learning. Jamie explained that they entered the programme with the idea that feminism was the movement of women taking power, and the need for a reimagining of women as being strong and able and not weak and vulnerable. They explained that this was met with the Intercordia invitation to live vulnerability in a way that interrogated this conception of feminism, and they began to ask whom this construction of feminism might marginalize or oppress. Jamie began to question how this might be an ableist construction of feminism and can work to further marginalize. Jamie explained that this analysis was enabled by the invitation to accept and embrace human vulnerability as a way of entering into more mutual and just relationships with the *other*. Jamie engaged in a difficult analysis that interrogated their own internalization of ableism, using vulnerability to push them into this difficult learning.

Vulnerability as Freedom

One student participant, Hunter, explained how they worked at unpacking the normative narratives of changing the world and the humanitarian imperative of the Northerners as helper (Heron, 2007). They said,

> I feel like, Intercordia it gives you the experience, it already gives you the whole vulnerability bit, in that, you know that you are not really capable. You can't be actively saying, "I gotta go out and make change, and it has to be me, and I have to go change things." So on one hand you can't really say that. On the other hand, you can't just dismiss it as an experience you had and it's over … Now that I've done it, I stay that it stays with me and it makes me want to have more. I had such strong relationships and connections with people that I met there, and I think that that is pretty great, and it, because of that, it makes it impossible for me to say it was just a learning experience and it's over. It has to be an on-going thing, that I am – and I want to continue.

Hunter struggled to think through what they wanted to say here and ended with "I don't think that I am going to go out and change the world or whatever. Cause I think Intercordia makes you think twice about having that sort of mentality." Here Hunter is engaged in disrupting the IESL constructions of the Northern helper (Jefferess, 2012). Their learning included naming their own vulnerability, their own littleness in the face of large structural problems that cannot be solved through the actions of the individual. I understand this as a freedom from these false and oppressive narratives; the fantasy that we can save or change the world, that the answer to structural problems is individual response. The reproduction of neoliberalism in this space; individuals must make change, not systems. Vrasti (2012) speaks to the participants' disillusionment with this desire to change the world, a desire that is bound to fail, leaving you empty and disempowered. The tools of capital cannot fix the contradictions of capitalism; volunteering abroad will not make the world a more just place. The call to embrace one's vulnerability, in contrast, is achievable. It takes self-reflexive processing work and time, which Hunter explains as a process of freedom, which was one that moved them to seek out a more authentic mutual relationship and connection. Here vulnerability was generative and emancipatory.

Vulnerable Mentors

I interviewed two student participants who later served as mentors for Intercordia, and both positioned the role of mentor as essential in supporting students in their learning and vulnerability. I asked them specific questions about their role as mentor, one rooted in the pedagogy of journeying with student participants, a call to be with student participants in their difficult learning, not moving to make their learning comfortable or easy (Intercordia, 2016). I was struck by the way the two mentors spoke about struggles and emotions that student participants lived, in very complex ways. There was no use of medicalized mental health language; no move to individualize what student participants were living. The mentors revealed their understanding of student participants' struggles as being a normal process, not as abnormal or stigmatized. One of the mentors, Kana, talked about their own struggles with change and living the experience well, and I was struck by their construction of struggle or anguish as normal and part of the human experience, and something that they wanted to strive to live well. Kana did not move to eliminate, fix, or avoid struggle, but instead committed to live it as well as they could. I understand this is an essential part of the model of support in Intercordia. Student participants are told that they will struggle, that they will live through difficult times, they will feel hopelessness and anguish, as this is a part of living with those experiencing poverty and structural violence (Intercordia, 2016). The call to participants is to work to live the experience in healthy ways, and to work to find ways to live through it with support and tools; mentorship, peer support, and tools like journaling (Intercordia, 2016). There is not a move to individualize anguish, the outside pressures and realities are acknowledged as well as the accepting of one's own embodied experience as part of the situation. There is a real danger here, that I identify, that the programming can be implemented as ableist, fitting into the larger critique of the international development field as not being inclusive of those who are unable to "tough it out." The larger criticism of social justice spaces as ableist is relevant here (Zaikowski, 2016).

Kana, a mentor, explained that they re-read their journal from their experience in preparation for our interview. They realized how difficult their first few days in placement were. They described their reaction after they arrived in their overseas placement:

Usually my reaction when travelling is that after the first couple of days, actually usually the first couple of hours, I will have a break-down. And that happened when I went. And it was one of my super vulnerable points ... Recognizing that that is how I travel. It happens every time.

Kana explained that they understood this as a normal reaction to cultural adjustment, and as wanting to share it with the student participants that they were supporting, as an intentional move to reveal their own vulner-ability. To create a space where student participants would feel comfortable sharing their own vulnerabilities. Kana talked about a moment of reading in their journal the following lines:

Didn't journal last night. Didn't want to be alone with my thoughts. And totally freaking out, right. So, um, being at least able to talk to somebody about it. Or just cry. And like, let something out, but not feel that weight of, of being isolated and alone.

Kana had a deep understanding of living in struggle as a subjective one, not a medicalized or pathologized objective one, and that they wanted to share it with student participants in order to normalize it. To invite them to feel what they are feeling and offer some suggestions of ways to respond and cope. Kana explained that their own experience opened them up to wanting to be with student participants in their low times. They revealed that they struggled with whether they should share the experience with the student participants, as they were there as a support to them, unsure of how such deep vulnerability would be read or received. But they explained that they reflected on this and decided that they wanted to be vulnerable with them. I understand this as a real moment of disrupting ideas of vulnerability, and who can and should be vulnerable in relations under capital. Those who hold power and authority do not make known their vulnerability. Those imagined as a source of support do not make known their anxieties or times of struggle. Kana, the mentor, made an intentional choice to be vulner-able with those she was supporting, as a method of being a more effective and empathetic mentor. A move to embody leadership in a different way, rooted in the Intercordia ethos of vulnerability enabling deeper relationships (Intercordia, 2016). When I asked Kana about a story of success, I heard more about their struggles with identifying as what one might see as suc-cessful in relations under capital. They said that looking back, they don't feel overly successful in their role as mentor, but is hopeful that the successes are there. For Kana, emotional success was important; the relationships that they helped mediate culturally and language-wise between hosts and student participants were moments of success. Kana named this as important labour they engaged in, work in engaging in the world otherwise, disrupting rela-tions structured under capital (Andreotti & DeSouza, 2012).

I want to end this section on student reflections on vulnerability with an attentiveness to ways this learning and pedagogy can perpetuate harm and reproduce capitalist power relations. Intercordia's pedagogical focus on vulnerability was one where vulnerability is a universal experience and one that can call us to deeper relationships of mutuality, which become a site where Northerners risk engaging in inaccurate or damaging learning. The risk becomes engaging in a learning that states: my vulnerability (shrouded or protected by privilege) is equal to your vulnerability as an oppressed or marginalized *other* under intersecting systems of colonialism, imperialism, and capitalism. This is not historically or materially accurate. And it can operate as a way to erase transnational historical, colonial, and material oppression. It can erase ways that Northern privilege operates, embedded in and produced by systems of domination and oppression. The emancipatory potential of the centring of vulnerability as a generative basis for encounters with the *other* is a learning that states: my own vulnerability has opened me up to accepting you, the *other,* as teacher, as knowledge-holder, as agent in your emancipation however you imagine and work towards that. A learning that states: my vulnerability has allowed me to occupy a critical, self-reflexive space that opens me up to processing and accepting my own role in your oppression. For undergraduate students from the North, this space is a difficult one to fully embrace or enter. And the pull to enter the first space of learning is strong, as it is comforting and affirming. Northern university students engaged in Intercordia through these narratives already known (Jefferess, 2013). An alternative program is not immune from the reproduction of these disabling narratives. The space of IESL is fraught with already known disabling narratives about those who deserve pity and those who can bestow this pity. A space that needs disruption, troubling and interventions; some would say abolition. Critical pedagogy and intention cannot guarantee the disruption of disablement; the danger of reproduction of disablement is always a possibility.

Pedagogical Invitations for Vulnerability

As educators, we must build alternatives, disruptions, within the growing uncritical IESL field, and create programmes that really challenge students, engage them to think critically, allow them to meet and understand those who are different on the terms of those from the South, and understand these encounters as existing in larger disabling systems. Opportunities to destabilize knowledge, ideas of and who can hold knowledge, and the creation of spaces to create new narratives for hope and a future resisting the project of dehumanizing neoliberalism is necessary work for educators to be actively engaging in. Vulnerability is a powerful pedagogical tool to enable this kind of deep decolonial learning, but must be done in spaces that are safe, critical, and supported in meaningful ways. The model of peer mentorship in Global South placement allows for this kind of deep learning using vulnerability, because the emotional labour is supported by peer mentors and does not fall (in its entirety) to Global South hosts, which happens in specific gendered and raced ways (Hernandez & Rerrie, 2018). What does a critical engagement with vulnerability look like in relations in our post- or with-COVID world, where inequities have been unveiled in deeper ways? Dionne Brand asks us to grapple with the fact that the "reckoning may be now" (2020, para. 9). A reckoning of the ways we have built our social relations, have built the world we have now. Brand urges us to grapple with this time of reckoning, as the window of time on our collective unmooring during pandemic times may close, and we need to take this time to engage in this time of unmooring to imagine and build the spaces we need to all thrive. How does this reckoning unfold in this space of learning and how can vulnerability engage us in different and more generative ways?

The stories of vulnerability taken up in this chapter provide us with examples of deep and rich learning that intervenes in the ableist and disabling narratives in mainstream IESL, troubling and complicating who knows, who helps, who should help, and why all of this is fraught and a space that needs a deep reckoning. When one engages with one's one vulnerability, in a safe and supportive educational space, the fertile ground to explore an unmooring of epistemological superiority and an openness to different ontologies and ways of being in the world become more possible. This engagement with vulnerability opens a space for students to sit and deeply engage with the openness to not knowing and to radically rethink about who knows, who holds knowledge, and who is in a position to teach and give. Vulnerability gave students a freedom from the colonial, from the ableist, from the damaging benevolent helper role that is so often reproduced in IESL encounters. While this chapter takes up the educational space of IESL, the employment of vulnerability as a pedagogical tool can be used in all education spaces. Really seeing, and welcoming, each student as they are, with their strengths and their vulnerabilities, is a gift that us educators can give those who come into our classrooms and educational spaces. Of course considerations of how this labour is gendered, raced, and disabled is something we must attend to, and it structures our ability, or inability, to do this work (Razack, 2001).

I began by asking the question: What does it mean to evoke mutuality within and against unequal power relations, between Southern hosts and Northern students in the space of international experiential service learning? The stories of vulnerability that students shared with me help us understand how they did the work of mutuality in these fraught neoliberal times. Perhaps what Dionne Brand (2020) is asking us to do is to reckon with our collective unmooring in generative ways, and a deep engagement with vulnerability as a pedagogical tool is part of how we can do this work together.

References

Andreotti, V. (2015). Global citizenship education otherwise: Pedagogical and theoretical insights. In A. Abdi, L. Shultz, & T. Pillay (Eds.), *Decolonizing global citizenship education* (pp. 221–230). Sense Publishers.

Andreotti, V., & de Souza, L. M. (2012). Introduction: (Towards) global citizenship education 'otherwise.' In V. Andreotti & L. M. de Souza (Eds.), *Postcolonial perspectives on global citizenship education* (pp. 1–6). Routledge.

Brand, D. (2020). On narrative, reckoning and the calculus of living and dying. July 4, 2020. *The Toronto Star*. Retrieved from https://www.thestar.com/ entertainment/books/2020/07/04/dionne-brand-on-narrative-reckoning-and-the -calculus-of-living-and-dying.html?rf

Chouliaraki, L. (2013). *The ironic spectator: Solidarity in the age of post-humanitarianism.* Polity Press.

Conran, M. (2011). They really love me!: Intimacy in volunteer tourism. *Annals of Tourism Research, 38*(4), 1454–1473. https://doi.org/10.1016/j.annals.2011.03 .014

Erevelles, N. (2000). Educating unruly bodies: Critical pedagogy, disability studies, and the politics of schooling. *Educational Theory, 50*(1), 25–47. https://doi.org/ 10.1111/j.1741-5446.2000.00025.x

Gorman, R. (2016). Disablement in and for itself: Towards a 'global' idea of disability. *Somatechnics, 6*(2), 249–261. https://doi.org/10.3366/soma.2016.0194

Grech, S., & Soldatic, K. (Eds.). (2016). *Disability in the global south: The critical handbook.* Springer.

Hernandez, X., & Rerrie, A. (2018). Where are the host mothers? How gendered relations shape the international experiential learning program experience for women in the south. *Journal of Global Citizenship and Equity Education, 6*(1). Retrieved from https://journals.sfu.ca/jgcee/index.php/jgcee/article/view/177

Heron, B. (2007). *Desire for development: The education of White women as development workers.* Wilfred Laurier University Press.

Huish, R., & Tiessen, R. (2014). Afterward: There should be nothing experimental about experiential learning: From globetrotting to global citizenship. In R. Tiessen & R. Huish (Eds.), *Globetrotting or global citizenship?: Perils and potential of international experiential learning* (pp. 280–287). University of Toronto Press.

Intercordia. (2016). Seminar book. Unpublished Internal document [PDF available upon request to chapter author].

Jefferess, D. (2012). Unsettling cosmopolitanism: Global citizenship and the cultural politics of benevolence. In V. Andreotti & L. M. de Souza (Eds.), *Postcolonial perspectives on global citizenship education* (pp. 27–46). Routledge.

Jefferess, D. (2013). Humanitarian relations: Emotion and the limits of critique. *Critical Literacy: Theories and Practices, 7*(1), 73–83. Retrieved from http://www .criticalliteracyjournal.org

Larkin, A. (2012). Implications for Canadian higher education internationalization policies: Critical considerations on the impact of the shift to knowledge exports from cooperative and development programming. *Potentia, 1*(4), 73–88. Retrieved from https://uottawa.scholarsportal.info/ottawa/index.php/potentia/ article/view/4396

MacDonald, K. (2016). *Pedagogical encounters and volunteer abroad in Nicaragua* [Unpublished doctoral dissertation]. University of Alberta.

MacDonald, K., & Vorstermans, J. (2015). Struggles for mutuality: Conceptualizing hosts as participants in international service learning in Ghana. In M. Larsen (Ed.), *International service learning: Engaging host communities* (pp. 131–146). Routledge.

Mahrouse, G. (2014). *Conflicted commitments: Race, privilege and power in transnational solidarity activism*. McGill-Queen's University Press.

Mostafanezhad, M. (2014). *Volunteer tourism: Popular humanitarianism in neoliberal times*. Ashgate.

Oliver, M. (1990). *The politics of disablement*. Macmillan Education.

Razack, N. (2001). Diversity and difference in the field education encounter: Racial minority students in the practicum. *Social Work Education, 20*(2), 220–232. https://doi.org/10.1080/02615470120044310

Shubert, A., Jones, G. A., & Desai Trilokekar, R. (2009) Introduction. In R. Desai Trilokekar, G. A. Jones, & A. Shubert (Eds.), *Canada's universities go global* (pp. 7–16). James Lorimer & Company Ltd.

Tiessen, R., & Epprecht, M. (2012). Introduction: Global citizenship education for learning/volunteering abroad. *Journal of Global Citizenship and Equity Education, 2*(1) (Special Edition), 1–11. Retrieved from https://journals.sfu.ca/jgcee/index.php/jgcee/article/view/54

Vorstermans, J. (2018a). Imagining, constructing and reifying disability in volunteer abroad: Able global citizens helping the disabled southern other. *Journal of Global Citizenship and Equity Education, 6*, 1. Retrieved from https://journals .sfu.ca/jgcee/index.php/jgcee/article/view/181

Vorstermans, J. (2018b). *Theorizing encounters with southern disabled others: The reproduction of disablement in international experiential service learning and global citizenship education and invitations for disruptions* [Unpublished doctoral dissertation]. York University.

Vrasti, W. (2012). *Volunteer tourism in the global South: Giving back in neoliberal times*. Routledge.

Zaikowski, C. (2016, September 20). 6 ways your social justice activism might be ableist. *Everyday Feminism*. Retrieved from http://everydayfeminism.com/2016 /09/social-justice-activism-ableist/

Part 2

Pedagogies of Overcoming Silence

Many reasons can contribute to silence about a traumatic event associated with pain and suffering. Some reasons include processing the emotions and feelings, silence for survival and as a coping mechanism, strategizing about how to respond and mobilize, or not finding a brave or supportive space to share. For example, in critiquing why many men grow up not sharing their feelings with their partners, in *All about Love: New Visions* bell hooks (2000) points out, "From the moment little boys are taught they should not cry or express hurt, feelings of loneliness, or pain, that they must be tough, they are learning how to mask true feelings" (p. 38). Overcoming silence and speaking up is at the core of healing, feeling empowered, and being confident and resilient to share the pain and suffering with intentionality. As Indigenous artist Lyla June reminds us in her song "Mamwlad" (https://www.youtube.com/watch?v=TeGLDwfrvb8), a song in honour of the 6 million to 9 million Indigenous women persecuted as witches in Europe, "Feeling is healing and this is why we remember their names. Feeling is healing and this is why we wash away the pain, so let it rain on this land." (June, 2018) Although silence can be interpreted as a passive or submissive stance, this is not always the case. You can be silent strategically as a form of resistance or subversion (Eizadirad & Portelli, 2018). As the famous poet Rumi reminds us, "Listen to silence. It has so much to say." Overall, pedagogies of overcoming silence are process oriented and about the complexities and nuances involved in transitioning from being silent to choosing to share with intentionality with consideration for when to share, where, with whom, and for what purposes. These processes have unique trajectories for everyone and should not be generalized, given that we all have unique identities and cope with stressors differently.

Fluctuations in feelings are part of the human experience and the trajectory of growing which allows for opposite feelings and a vast range of emotions to be experienced, particularly how to embrace each emotion and what it can teach (#GiftofPain). When you decide whether to share your pain and suffering or remain in silence, you might grapple with the following questions: Do you feel safe in telling your story? Who will believe you? Who will support you? Is there trust? In what setting should you share?

DOI: 10.4324/9781003205296-6

Should you share in person or via an online platform? What medium should you use as a platform for your sharing? How are you impacted by sharing and how will others be impacted by listening? What consequences may arise from your sharing? These are questions you would engage with as you reflect, strategize, and mobilize about how to overcome silence as part of healing and as a form of activism and community advocacy.

It takes time, maturity, growth, and access to mentors and support networks to revisit traumatic experiences associated with pain and suffering to grapple with them constructively: to work with them and through them instead of choosing to forget or dismiss them. The process of sharing can occur in many ways and via various outlets and mediums. Some examples include sharing circles, journaling, poetry, drama and theatre, social media posts, spoken word performances, and paintings or drawings. In more recent years, advances in technology and the rise of popular social media platforms, such as Facebook, Twitter, TikTok, and Instagram, have made it easier to generate content and access it globally as part of online communities and networks. For some, due to their identity and social location, online platforms have made it easier to share their pain or the suffering of their community, at times anonymously due to safety reasons. These platforms have also been used to mobilize communities for collective resistance, hence why some countries have banned such platforms as means of silencing criticism. Online platforms can provide a means for counternarratives to be shared by authentic voices instead of others in positions of power speaking on behalf of oppressed groups. As a famous African proverb states, "Until lions have their own historians, tales of the hunt shall always glorify the hunter," meaning those in power can influence how the story is told, in the process selectively emphasizing what is important and what is left out.

Overcoming silence and sharing via storytelling is a powerful act. Oral traditions and passing of intergenerational knowledges are integral to many cultures and practices in the world, particularly in the Middle East, Africa, and with Indigenous ways of life. Overcoming silence, at times within our own imagination and thoughts, is an important prerequisite advancing towards sharing the pain with others in a way that is healing and transformative. It is a powerful experience to hone and own your story. It takes time, patience, and practice. As Woodfox (2019), who spent 40 years in solitary confinement, emphasizes, "We had been through so much brutality, so much pain and suffering that we had every right to be hard, bitter, and hateful towards almost everyone and everything in life. But instead, we did not allow prison to shape us. We defined ourselves" (p. 199). Woodfox further discusses how he capitalized on the agency he had while surviving under oppressive jail conditions that challenged him physically, socially, emotionally, and psychologically: "My proudest achievement in all my years in solitary was teaching a man how to read" (p. 163).

As we further engage with pedagogies of overcoming silence, it is important to reflect on the following questions: In any given situation, who benefits from the silence? Is sharing multiple perspectives encouraged or leads to repercussions? What has contributed systemically to many Black, Indigenous, and People of Colour (BIPOC) continuing to be silent about their negative experiences within educational contexts? How can we help others overcome silence as a form of unlearning? What processes exist that encourage sharing of narratives associated with pain and suffering? How are such narratives received and has it led to any changes or outcomes at the institutional level? We need to invest in processes that facilitate overcoming silence to present authentic voices and narratives to help others unlearn and advance equity and social justice. This is messy work that is not linear, yet it has the potential to be therapeutic and transformative. Overcoming silence and telling and reliving trauma as critical pedagogy is a counternarrative that disrupts and dispels deficit thinking and stereotypical representations. Sharing the pain and suffering as a form of calculated risk-taking, where negative emotions and feelings are harnessed constructively, becomes a skill and a form of strength rather than a weakness.

References

Eizadirad, A., & Portelli, J. (2018). Subversion in education: Common misunderstandings and myths. *International Journal of Critical Pedagogy*, *9*(1), 53–72.

hooks, b. (2000). *All about love: New visions.* Harper Perennial.

June, L. [Lyla June] (2018, May 3). *Lyla June – Mamwlad official video* [Video]. YouTube. Retrieved from https://www.youtube.com/watch?v=TeGLDwfrvb8

Woodfox, A. (2019). *Solitary: Unbroken by four decades in solitary confinement. My story of transformation and hope.* Harper Collins.

5 Co-Composing Poetic and Arts-Based Narratives

Un-Silencing and Honouring Our Voices as Women Academics

Anita Lafferty and Julie A. Mooney

Rising Voices

We are two women scholars, one Dene/Cree and one Irish-Scottish Canadian, inquiring into our experiences of being silenced in educational institutions and how we recover our voices. We use poetic and arts-informed methods to (re)signify, (re)captivate, and (re)identify with our shared and differed experiences of silencing. As women scholars, we attend to our poetic and artful voices to reflect our "identity negotiation processes, to question traditional representations of marginalized identities" (Faulkner, 2009, p. 29). In answering the call to engage with *pain and suffering*, we establish the commonality of our experiences as often abrupt silencing.

Un-silencing is a taking back of our voices in the places we felt voiceless; this work is a *voicing of self*. In this chapter, we focus on the question asked by Sameshima and colleagues (2018), "How might poetic inquiry [and arts] encourage texts that illustrate possibilities, advocate for silenced voices, and address challenges and tensions?" (p. 18). Within these spaces that often silence our voices, how might we ethically and in *good relations,* unpack our lived experiences of pain and suffering? Good relations refer to connecting as though we are relatives and honouring each other's voices as equal. In Cree, the word that relays this is *wicihitowin* (Donald, 2016, p. 10). Collectively, we must begin to change the narratives from male-dominated to include women's stories and voices equally. Our stories hold significance, our histories hold truth, and our voices hold agency. As our experiences unfold the complexities of being silenced, we become wakeful to "what it is to be in the world" as women scholars and to pay attention to silences as we question power relations (Greene, 1995, p. 35). There is space for our voices to come together in harmony when we *all* – people of all genders – listen and *act* collectively as advocates for change.

Poetic rhythms and the emotions evoked by poetry invite the reader-listener into holistic and embodied ways of knowing (Butler-Kisber, 2010). It is this embodiment that moves us into a space where our voices freely formulate the realities of our experiences. Faulkner (2009) explains that the "embodied experience recognizes the need for poetry to make audiences feel

DOI: 10.4324/9781003205296-7

with, rather than *about* a poem, to experience emotions and feeling in situ" (p. 90). As Indigenous and non-Indigenous scholars, we found commonalities and differences in our writings about our silences. Our connection to poetry prompted our responses, as Lorde (2017) explains: "Poetry is not only the dream and vision; it is the skeleton architecture of our lives" (p. 9). We dream of equality and shared understandings, a wider-reaching space of ethical relations, where our voices are expressed and heard. Our vision is to share our experiences in ways that recognize, reverberate, render, rivet, roar, and rise with other women. This vision, enacted together, is a form of critical pedagogy – a way of learning that repudiates supremacy, restores justice, reclaims agency, and honours relationality.

As we reveal our lived experiences, we recognize that "we must put ourselves in the context; we must feel, taste, hear what someone is saying [or not saying] … We must be empathetic, aware, non-judgemental, and cautious" (Pendergast, 2009, p. xxvi). Cautious so we do not resettle with the pain and suffering; cautious in our words so we do not distort the narratives or have them hold onto us as defining. We found that by embracing poetry a art, we can respond to the silencing overtly while "living ethically as a researcher in the field" (Leggo et al., 2011, p. 244). The use of poetic inquiry and arts-based research, for us, functions as a counternarrative to the dominant voices that disregard or are seemingly unaware of the silences we experience. In order to prioritize our individual voices and attend to each other relationally, we shape and (re)shape our stories back and forth under four headings: experiencing being silenced, coming to know our voices, speaking to and from our heart voices, and attending to our voices. We do this to draw into our words and experiences and "call forth the embodied responses within us" (Clandinin et al., 2018, p. 157).

Experiencing Being Silenced

Anita's Narrative

> *silence* is both a verb and a noun,
> a subject and a predicate:
> silence silences
>
> (Leggo, 2009, p. 159)

My story is about how curriculum has silenced me throughout my many years of being a student. I am Dene and Cree, and I grew up not seeing the beauty of Indigenous women's history within the context of my education. Sadly, not much has changed. It is difficult to feel silenced in education. Curriculum silenced me as an Indigenous person and education silenced me as a Dene Cree. It left me rendered quiet within the history books, within the complex conversations, within the coursework, and within the subject matter. The pedagogy of my ancestral knowledge was not found within the context of my learning landscapes. If it was found, it was rare and felt as though my tongue was stripped from my mouth declaring me silent. It was the abrupt silences that often kept me from embracing my identity as a *ts'élî iskwew*.[1] The lack of Indigenous identity within curriculum ultimately undermined what generations of matriarchs were prohibited to teach me while leaving me to (re)learn culture and language.

The silence of Indigenous matriarchal history and the silence of being a First Nation woman is not only profound but difficult to process at times. I pause and reflect on the closed conscientiousness of my teachers, administrators, and policymakers, and I wonder how they decided "what knowledge is of most worth" to teach (Pinar, 2012, p. xv). I have learned many stories of strong women in my community and even more within the wider context of Indigenous communities throughout Canada. It comes as no surprise that "Western culture has typically not promoted, documented or explored the culture(s) of its women" (Anderson, 2016, p. 30). There is resistance to what we deem as *progress* for women while oppressive and colonial systems still dominate. It is time to question colonial intelligence and critique the accounts of history in curriculum, knowing that "to hold alternative histories is to hold alternative knowledges [which gives access] to alternative ways of doing things" (Smith, 2012, p. 36). Coming to know theory and research from a Dene Cree matriarchal lens allows me to understand history in the way it was intended, with Indigenous voices as core history offering valuable perspectives and purpose to my epistemological foundation as a Dene Cree woman.

I Wonder

jarring voices dominating the narrative
I wonder if my story could exist

resilient powerful voice; still silenced!
I wonder if they hear me

blurred vision shapes a foggy landscape ahead
I wonder if they imagine my ancestors as mythical

no comment, no movement, no reconciliation
I wonder if my sister comrades hear them too

thunderous women as counternarratives in strong stories
I wonder when the dominant stories will be rewritten to include ours.

I echo the words of Anderson (2016), Simpson (2013), Maracle (1996), Armstrong (1996), and many other Indigenous women scholars, who recognize and honour matriarchal ways within pedagogical practices as a way to return to the grandmothers. I am not alone in the silences; we have all endured within this Western context. It is a time for transformation, it is time to act. Through poetry and expressions of art I am able to find ways to recontextualize, be diligent with my words, (de)construct, and (re)construct pedagogy as a place to tell truths.

Un-silence Ama[2]

instinct will tell you how to live your life
rise with your purpose
womanhood nurtured me
the Earth mother, the sacredness embodied within
spiritual notions metamorphosizes my blood memory

but I am still found compelled by colonial dispositions
as the dark shadows in the bleak pages of the past
where the beautiful lives of femme were torn from the histories
riddled with despair
the fight we encounter, still,
is like a fight with giants
the feeling
like we; the matriarchs, the mothers, the sisters, the aunties, the relatives
so small. so minute. so invisible.

it is the conscious awakening that becometh me
seeping through the edge of desire
desire to walk in balance
desire to float into the abyss
as a flux in nature
unravelling the layers idling in fear

such disgrace and injustice that we are still
negotiating boundaries of existence
like fallacy of fallacies unravelling in mummified form
ancient teachings lost in the abyss
due to lack of acknowledgement
of existence of reverence of phenomenality
bequeath my soul for this state of emergency
is rampant in my mind
resist the query into the silence – behold the matriarch rising!

From this poem, I created a collage reflecting on the metaphor of silence. Through this process, I explored where the curriculum of silence is situated.

Captured is the imagery of silenced matriarchal voices, the silence of Indigenous voices, and the image of where the language is situated but found invisible and silent upon my tongue. Davis and Butler-Kisber (1999) explain that "the collage process helps suspend linear thinking and allow elusive qualities of feelings and experiences to be addressed tangibly" (p. 1). As I think about the colonial misguidance of matriarchal voices, the images within this collage began to emerge. I sought to portray the galvanized displacement of matriarchs throughout history. Mother Earth (Ama; my mother) is placed centrally, as it is central to the teachings and the Cree and Dene languages I am (re)learning. My mother is my first teacher, the core of the Earth. The surrounding images relay the context of what has been missing in my lived experiences of education, history, media, languages, and curriculum. It magnifies the fact that matriarchal voices and, even further than that, Indigenous voices have been absent from historical narratives that I have and continue to encounter (Figure 5.1).

Julie's Narrative

As a settler Canadian woman of Irish-Scottish ancestry, I have worked as an educational developer and a teacher in higher education for over a decade. I am currently working on my PhD in educational policy studies with a focus on how university professors are learning to indigenize and decolonize their teaching and curricular practices. Not wanting to perpetuate the silencing and erasure, I work to open space for and listen to Indigenous voices in the communities of learners alongside which I teach and learn. As an ongoing process, I aim to disrupt and unsettle my colonial assumptions and mindset (Regan, 2010).

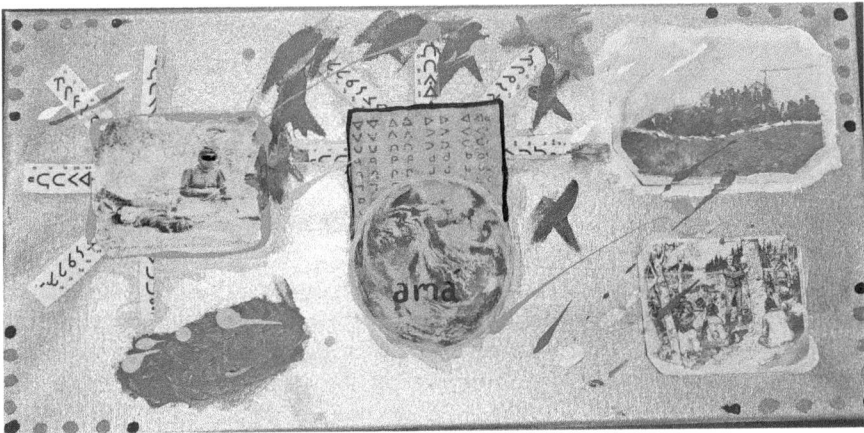

Figure 5.1 Where Matriarch Voices Were Silenced [collage], by A. Lafferty, 2021.

Western neoliberal academic institutions are highly hierarchical and patriarchal spaces (Carter & Janes, 2018). While I benefit from white privilege and colonialism, as a woman doctoral student, I am relatively low ranking in academic hierarchies. I have been silenced and sidelined. Most often, but not always, it has been other women who have exerted dominance to render me silent. I felt especially betrayed when women in positions of authority not only failed to mentor me, but actively worked to break me, whether intentionally or not. I wonder what happened to sister solidarity (Lyle, 2020), as hooks (2003a) reminds us that "sexism pits women against one another" (p. 61). Lateral and top-down forms of violence between women are prominent in academic spaces, and they carry the hidden practices of competition, grudges, and favouritism. My experiences of being silenced often happened in private meetings with no witnesses to attest to acts of aggression, such as threats of punishment, personal insults, and gaslighting.

Words that Silenced Me

"Try not to be so feminist, so out-spoken!"
"Don't bother requesting a transfer, I'm the only one willing to work with you"
"Well, aren't you clever? Be careful not to make your colleagues look bad."
when they fail to break me
they ask, with envy and suspicion:
"How do you do it? Stay so composed?,"
but my lack of tears in those moments was not for lack of pain
I felt deeply disappointed
a sense of loss, a sense of grief,
why is it so difficult to find a woman mentor,
an academic auntie,
a sister scholar,
to support my growth
to be a champion for my journey in academia?

It is disheartening to experience these aggressive expressions of domination that permeate educational institutions, silencing and causing harm to those either in subordinate positions or perceived to be somehow subordinate.[3] Carter and Janes (2018) explain that women, transitioning in workplaces, especially within leadership positions "often encounter difficult and demoralizing circumstances" (p. 210). Bullying and abuse of power often mask the perpetrator's own experiences of oppression and struggles to be heard. Those who have a history of being bullied or marginalized are more likely to become bullies if they have a high level of self-esteem (Choi & Park, 2018). Those who are targeted by bullying are more likely to respond passively and avoid resisting when they value collectivism over individualism and have a high-power distance[4] (Ólafsson & Jóhannsdóttir, 2004; Samnani, 2013). In the experiences I have explored in the preceding poem, not only was I silenced, but I was separated from a community of colleagues – the collective. Being silenced and alienated, by individuals with power over me, communicated that my voice was unwelcome, that I did not belong in those academic circles.

Silence Ruptured

when I finally met a woman supervisor in academia
who treated me with respect and dignity,
who was honest and shared her knowledge freely,
who listened to me, and valued my contributions,
I was brought to tears,
tears of relief and release
from the pain of silencing
I have experienced over many years,
across educational contexts.
What is it about some women in positions of power?
Why is their violence so common, cruel, and hostile?
What happens to women following in their footsteps?
Why are generous women mentors not the norm?

Emphasis on Our Voices

Anita's Narrative

Basso (1996) explains that wisdom sits in place. It is formed through careful attention to place, relationship, and story. In my school experiences, not all places of learning were honoured as wisdom. "The important value of non-verbal communication beneath language" (Lorde, 2007, p. 83) is like the silent teachings my mother taught me. I learned by listening, by watching, and by observing. Oftentimes there were no directives of right or wrong, there was only guidance in movements of the silent walks. There were the many stories shared among aunties as I learned by being and doing along-side my matriarchs. As a student, I used these same skills in the classroom. I listened. I watched. And I observed. When I did not like what I heard in school, I bit my tongue and silently raged against the colonial patriarchy forcefully staring me down. Now, as a doctoral student, I continue to (re)envision, (re)establish, and (re)negotiate curriculum, forming alternative ways of knowing that include the voices of my matriarchs.

Where the Wisdom Lives

wisdom lives with the matriarchs
        as they share their light & visions for walking as strong women

wisdom lives in the lines of my grandmother's face
>> the beauty of her soul is present in her strong hands that have
>> and still carry me
wisdom lives in the presence of ancestors found upon Mother Earth
>> where our roots are spread throughout the Land
wisdom lives in the stories of the grannies
>> their strength, courage, determination & reverence exist within
>> us all
wisdom lives where the silences have formed
>> as their voices are heard in the whispers of the treetops
wisdom lives with the elements of "being and doing"
>> as strong matriarchs emerge throughout the world
wisdom lives with the teachings of ancient wisdom
>> as the stories engage spirit and transfer the old ways forward
wisdom lives within the spirit of my daughter
>> as she stands for the generations of matriarchs to come
wisdom lives within us, strong women, formulating our voices
>> to be spoken, to be heard, and to be honoured

Julie's Narrative

To recover after jolting experiences of being silenced, I often go for a walk outdoors. The healing properties of movement in a natural setting have been well documented; among the benefits one can reap are reduced stress and anxiety, relief from depression, and increased creative thinking (Berman, Jonides, & Kaplan, 2008; Oppezzo & Schwartz, 2014; Selhub & Logan, 2012). On one particular day, I went for a walk under the wide-open sky, where tall grasses and prairie crocuses grow wildly. I sought solace in solitude along the river. I ached with longing for belonging, for a place where my voice would be heard and honoured.

As I walked, I arrived at a stretch of land where prairie grasses had been recently burned. The dramatic blackened landscape was speckled with tiny bright green shoots of new growth –signs of hope. Having been burned by silencing in educational institutions, when the burns healed, from the ashes of that fire would sprout new growth in me. Out on the land, I could put myself back together again and imagine myself whole, with my breath restored and my voice alive. That walk gave me hope, it helped me recover my sense of self, remembering that my voice matters, and I have much to contribute (Figures 5.2 and 5.3).

Prairie Burning

wind sweeping pain
that sears my skin and calls my name
the heart catches fire

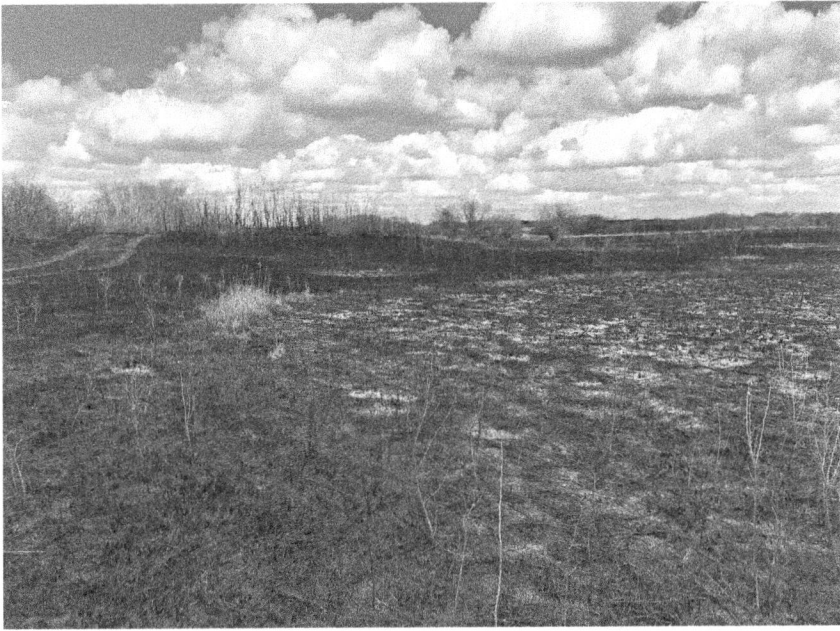

Figure 5.2 Prairie Burning 1 & 2 [photograph], by J. A. Mooney, 2019.

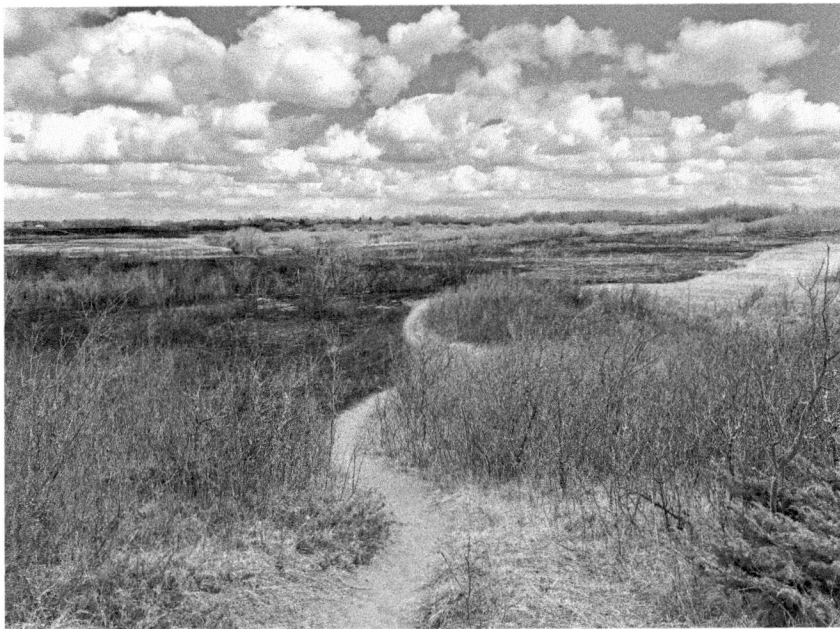

Figure 5.3 Prairie Burning 1 & 2 [photograph], by J. A. Mooney, 2019.

like the prairie grasses
where I walk
one foot in front of the next
one step at a time

breath taken; voice shaken
grief and rage stir these guts
how many times must I turn another page?
unwelcomed by the mighty few
I start anew

I'm the one who carves my path
the narrator of my own story
tangled up with so many stories
generations of wrongs, shameful
historical treaties and current day dealings
I work to dismantle systems that wound
and pray that I too may endure this pain
without turning sour

walking along the river
one step at a time
one foot in front of the next
small steps, taken often;[5] persistently
bring change.

Speaking to and from Our Heart Voices

Anita's Narrative

"Women will starve in silence, until new stories are created which confer on them the power of naming themselves and controlling their world" (Gilbert et al., 2020, p. 391) articulates the necessity for stories of, about, and for women, by women. Although Julie's and my stories differ, there are healing qualities revealed in our truths. As we begin to challenge the dominant narratives and shift the heteropatriarchal ideologies that exist within educational spaces, collectively our stories hold power. We are creating space for new narratives to emerge within these boundaries and evading the conformity. Figure 5.4 is of a painted stone art piece I created. The painting is focused on strong matriarchal words that confer the power of women. Words such as strength, love, guzhǫ (wise), story tellers, dįį ndéh (earth), ǫdze (moon), rootedness, gogha goenehté (teacher), healing, and sisterhood. These are words that, for me, prioritize matriarchal voices. Words that are found in the oral histories, words that hold social power, words that determine our

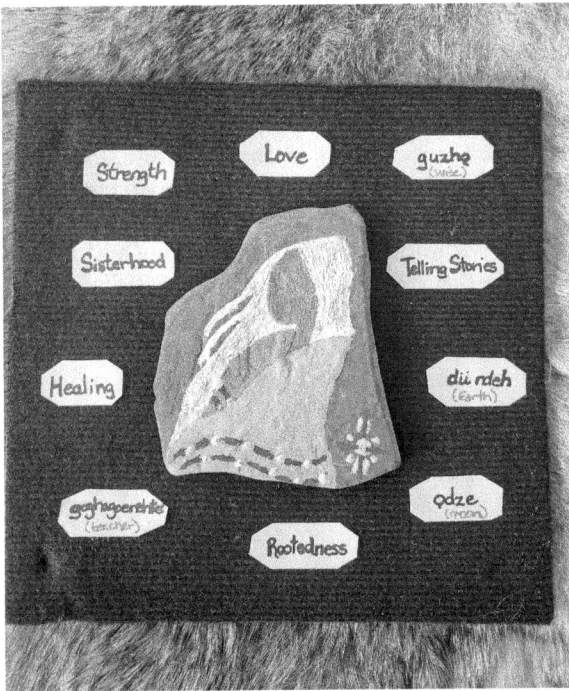

Figure 5.4 Matriarchal Perspectives, [painted stone art piece], by A. Lafferty, 2021.

matrilineal society, words that speak to leadership, and words that speak to honour.

> *In Looking Forward I See*
> historical photographs reveal
>> the dynamic strength of Indigenous matriarchs
>> strong voices heard
>> and revered as offerings to be honoured
> the languages emerge from the tongues of the young ones
>> wisdom of the Land will shed light
>> on generations of knowledge keepers; rightfully so.
> sturdy hands will continue to take care of our needs,
>> with warming heart knowledge at the core
>> deep values summoned forth in royal form
>> as celebratory cheers radiate the authentic voices of women
> uplifting, uprising, upheld where the context of matriarchal futurisms
>> emerge, explode, engage, evade, exude, and excite
>> feminine rising, I see it now.

Julie's Narrative

Ultimately, the silencing I have experienced in unhealthy, unwelcoming educational spaces has contributed to my chosen departure from those places to seek new, safer circles where my voice is received with respect. I am the first woman and the first person in my family of origin to pursue a PhD. As I approach the completion of this significant milestone in my life, I feel supported by the love and pride my family members and ancestors have for me. They value and honour education, and I have drawn strength from them as I faced silencing experiences within academia. Seeking out and finding caring mentors has also been vital to my survival and success. These mentors – both peers and superiors – have become part of my academic family; they have helped me navigate some tough terrain. I choose to follow in the footsteps of academics who have nurtured my journey, creating safe, welcoming spaces in which I have been able to develop my research, teaching, and curricular practices and to emerge in my identity as a strong woman scholar (Figure 5.5).

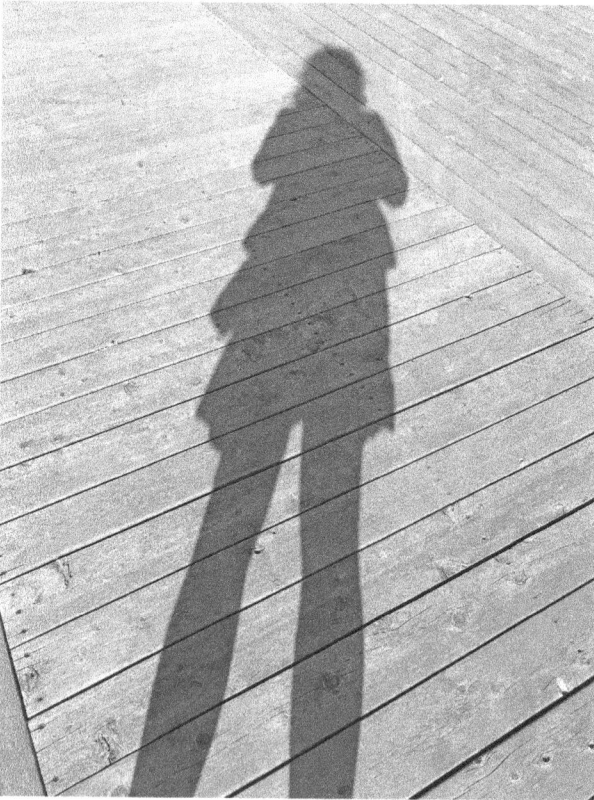

Figure 5.5 Shadow of Myself, No More [photograph], by J. A. Mooney, 2019.

Shadow of Myself, No More

crisp air
heavy heart
cerulean sky
unflinching sun
casts a shadow of myself
alienated, unwelcome
silenced
sidelined
I don't belong in isolation

I am a mountain, one of many
my heart beats
to mountain time
my voice rises at dawn
bounces along rock faces
dances in gorges
floats on misty waterfalls
skips atop canopies of evergreens
thunders through glacial rivers

pity the power-hungry
the egotistical
the aggressively insecure
the shameless bullies
who view me as a threat,
a competitor
shame on hierarchy, patriarchy,
any system that
divides and dehumanizes

pushed away
into the margins, onto the land
I hear my own voice, clearly
high noon
no shadow cast
fierce mountain woman
blazes new trail.

Attending to Our Voices

Julie's Narrative

Academic aunties[6] support women in the academy; they are trustworthy –
no games, no competition, no tests. They give women in academia courage

to be ourselves; to endure sexism, patriarchy, misogyny, and other oppressive structures; and to transform deficit narratives that hold us back from reaching our highest heights, where we are meant to soar, in all our phenomenality! By writing and voicing my counternarratives, I hope to transform myself and to help change the academy from within, one small act of un-silencing at a time.

Decolonizing teaching and learning cultures will require a wholesale change of academic institutions (Gaudry & Lorenz, 2018). Engaged in unlearning the settler colonial bias that has pervaded my education, I am working to re-educate myself (Mooney, 2021a, 2021b, 2021c; Tangney, Mooney & López Vélez, 2021), as best I can from an outsider position (Kuokkanen, 2007), to learn about Indigenous ways of knowing, and to build renewed, respectful, reciprocal relationships[7] alongside Indigenous colleagues, students, and community members, as we co-create a new, living curriculum (Aoki, 1993; Magrini, 2015) in postsecondary education.

I am grateful for communities of care (Southern, 2007) that gather around, as I continue to un-silence my stories. Attending to voice is rooted in a commitment to trust myself, my intuition, and my integrity as a women scholar. Innately relational, people of all genders thrive when we belong (Brown, 2007). The instinct of community is not uniquely human; "look at the evolutionary record, it is cooperation that increases over time. [...] nothing can exist without the other" (Wheatley, 2007, p. 47). I honour the land that nurtures me, helps me to attend to my voice, heals my brokenness, and restores my hope. Our institutions of higher learning need to acknowledge and embody that we are all interconnected and interdependent with one another and the land. To thrive as learning organizations, we must honour our need for connection, value each of our unique gifts, prioritize cooperation, and support one another's growth. While "building of healthy culture is an incremental process, with few shortcuts" (Carter & Janes, 2018, p. 224), these fundamental changes in academic culture are necessary to influence change in teaching and learning practices (Figure 5.6).

Place to Belong

sun and cold descending in the mountains
river carving path from icy elevations
I am learning to flow in harsh conditions,
I have returned to my beloved
this land, this place, this mountain range
embrace me, empower me, embolden me

I pay attention to the land
listen to the wind[8]
my heart is steady here
I breathe with ease

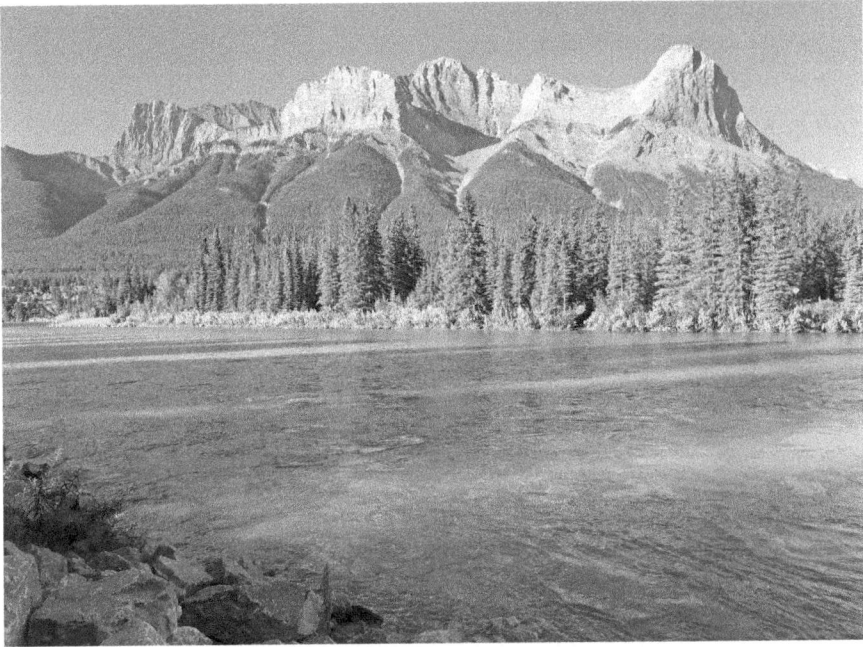

Figure 5.6 Place to Belong [photograph], by J. A. Mooney, 2020.

this is a welcoming
home, for now

my voice rises,
sings, grows quiet
I find superiors who question hierarchy
they encourage me when I stumble,
growing in their care, learning in community
accompanying one another
no judgement wielded
no reprisal, I receive
gentle nudges, loving guidance
I trust them with my true self

reciprocally, responsibly, relationally,[9]
understanding my privilege
building respectful relationship
mediating belonging,
in these unceded treaty lands
a settler Canadian,

a modern nomad[10]
creating an academic life
across diverse territories

Anita's Narrative

Words Without Voice

words that live in these stories and experiences
speak to no tone, they are voiceless words

what evokes pain you ask?
discrimination, dissemination, degradation
silences & muffled voices found in the background
set as an enigma, just for show

what provokes our voices?
utter disenchantment discovered in the cracks
hidden but absurdly unwelcomed by patriarchy
where are the male voices supporting us?
often rare in form or lost in translation

what stokes the fire from within?
ancient matriarchal voices,
the fighters, the warriors that lead the way
we stand united
withstanding the elements that keep us subdued

As we emerge into our voices poetically, we carefully listen to each other's lived experiences. We recognize similarities and differences. As we continue to think with stories of lived experience, we are living out new possibilities to reposition our voices within dominant narratives, to transform dominant histories, and to sideline ascendancy. We are contributing to the creation of space for women in the academy to attend to their own stories. Healing, for us, involves supporting each other, nurturing our voices as strong women, and co-composing counternarratives that allow us to stay wakeful as women scholars in unfamiliar and unwelcoming spaces.

The Land has been at the heart of the process for each of us, so we pay special attention to these lived experiences. As we trace the complexities of the pain and suffering and navigate the systemic oppressions that we both encounter as women, we find solace in our shared understandings. We are wakeful to our stories. We honour our voices as women scholars. Speaking our truth, not only as scholars but as women, is integral as we move to engage others who are coming into their voices or finding a place for their voice to be heard. As we thoughtfully find ways to support and encourage one another, our experiences bring forward a critical pedagogy through this practice of co-composing our storied lives. This practice incorporates critical hope (Regan, 2010) in community (hooks, 2003b) and relational ethics (Clandinin, Caine, & Lessard, 2018) in a process of caring for and attending to our own and each other's lived experiences.

By unravelling the complexities of our experiences as women in the academy, we attended to the voicing of self and paid "attention to those voices we have been taught to distrust, that we articulate what they teach us, that we act upon what we know" (Lorde, 2007, p. 12) in order to move forward with *wicihitowin*, in a good way. In this work we nurtured our understanding as women knowing that through our resilience, resurgence, and relationality, we co-composed poetic narratives of possibility. We found balance in our work together as two dynamic women scholars from two different places.

Matriarch Movement

WE are coming into balance
in relation; *wicihitowin*[11]
all voices honored
all voices recognized
where advocacy and agency elegantly collide
into powered energies of
truth, respect, and reclamation.
where patriarchy and matriarchy,
sing in harmony.
where we collectively locate
beautiful humanizing spaces
WE are coming into balance.

Notes

1 *Ts'éli* is Dene Zhatié for "woman." *Iskwew* is Plains Cree for "woman."
2 *Ama* is Dene Zhatié for "mother."
3 The hierarchy falsely assumes that some people are superior while some are subordinate.
4 "High power distance" refers to a greater distance on the hierarchy between bullying perpetrator and victimized (Hofstede et al., 2002).
5 "Small steps, taken often" (Colin Hunter in Rundle, 2019, minute 8:06).
6 Academic aunties grew out of Black, Indigenous, and People of Colour (BIPOC) communities in academia. They are akin to the cool aunt, but academic aunties are intentionally on a mission. See Curnow Wilson (2017). See also https://www.academicaunties.com.
7 See Kirkness and Barnhardt's (1991) four Rs theory.
8 "If we listen, nature will teach us" (hooks, 2009a, p. 25).
9 Kirkness and Barnhardt (1991).
10 "As a modern nomad, I do not stay in one place" (hooks, 2009b, p. 151).
11 Donald (2016).

References

Anderson, K. (2016). *A recognition of being: Reconstructing native womanhood.* Canadian Scholars' Press.

Aoki, T. (1993). Legitimating lived curriculum: Towards a curricular landscape of multiplicity. *Journal of Curriculum and Supervision, 8*(3), 255–268.

Armstrong, J. (1996). Aboriginal women. In C. Miller & P. M. Chuchryk (Eds.), *Women of the first nations: Power, wisdom, and strength* (pp. ix–xii). University of Manitoba Press.

Basso, K. H. (1996). *Wisdom sits in places: Landscape and language among the Western Apache.* UNM Press.

Berman, M. G., Jonides, J., & Kaplan, S. (2008). The cognitive benefits of interacting with nature. *Psychological Science, 19*(12), 1207–1212. https://doi.org/10.1111/j.1467-9280.2008.02225.x

Brown, B. (2007). *I thought it was just me (but it isn't): Making the journey from "what will people think?" to "I am enough".* Avery.

Butler-Kisber, L. (2010). Poetic inquiry. In *Qualitative inquiry: Thematic, narrative, and arts-informed perspectives* (pp. 82–98). SAGE Publications. Editor: Lynn Butler-Kisber

Carter, L. M., & Janes, D. P. (2018). The transition of women to leadership in post-secondary institutions in Canada: An examination of the literature and the lived DIM experiences of two female leaders. In C. Cho, J. Corkett, & A. Steele (Eds.), *Exploring the toxicity of lateral violence and microaggressions* (pp. 209–230). Palgrave Macmillan. https://doi.org/10.1007/978-3-319-74760-6

Choi, B., & Park, S. (2018). Who becomes a bullying perpetrator after the experience of bullying victimization? The moderating role of self-esteem. *Journal of Youth and Adolescence, 47*(11), 2414–2423.

Clandinin, D. J., Caine, V., & Lessard, S. (2018). *The relational ethics of narrative inquiry.* Routledge.

Curnow Wilson (2017 July 6). Cool aunts of academia. Connected Academics: Preparing doctoral students of language and literature for a variety of careers. https://connect.mla.hcom monss.org/cool-aunts-of-academia/

Davis, D., & Butler-Kisber, L. (1999, April). Arts-based representation in qualitative research: Collage as a contextualizing analytic strategy [Paper presentation]. American Educational Research Association annual meeting, Montreal, Canada. (ERIC Document Retrieval Service No. ED 431 790).

Donald, D. (2016). Chapter three: From what does ethical relationality flow? An "Indian" act in three artifacts. *Counterpoints, 478*, 10–16.

Faulkner, S. L. (2009). *Poetry as method: Reporting research through verse.* Left Coast Press.

Gaudry, A., & Lorenz, D. (2018). Indigenization as inclusion, reconciliation, and decolonization: Navigating the different visions for indigenizing the Canadian Academy. *AlterNative: An International Journal of Indigenous Peoples, 14*(3), 218–227.

Gilbert, S., Gubar, S., & Appignanesi, L. (2020). The genesis of hunger according to Shirley. In *The madwoman in the attic: The woman writer and the nineteenth-century literary imagination* (pp. 372–398). Yale University Press. https://doi.org/10.2307/j.ctvxkn74x.15

Greene, M. (1995). *Releasing the imagination: Essays on education, the arts, and social change*. Jossey-Bass.

Hofstede, G. J., Pedersen, P., & Hofstede, G. H. (2002). *Exploring culture: Exercises, stories, and synthetic cultures*. Nicholas Brealey Publishing.

hooks, b. (2003a). What happens when white people change (Chapter 5). In bell hooks (Ed.), *Teaching community: A pedagogy of hope* (pp. 51–66). Routledge.

hooks, b. (2003b). Keepers of hope: Teaching in communities (Chapter 9). In *Teaching community: A pedagogy of hope* (pp. 105–116). Routledge.

hooks, b. (2009a). *Belonging: A culture of place*. Routledge.

hooks, b. (2009b). Moved by mountains (Chapter 3). In bell hooks (Ed.), *Belonging: A culture of place* (pp. 25–33). Routledge.

Kirkness, V., & Barnhardt, R. (1991). First nations and higher education: The four Rs – Respect, relevance, reciprocity, and responsibility. *Journal of American Indian Education*, *30*(3), 9–16.

Kuokkanen, R. (2007). *Reshaping the university: Responsibility, indigenous epistemes, and the logic of the gift*. UBC Press.

Leggo, C., Sinner, A. E., Irwin, R. L., Pantaleo, K., Gouzouasis, P., & Grauer, K. (2011). Lingering in liminal spaces: A/r/tography as living inquiry in a language arts class. *International Journal of Qualitative Studies in Education*, *24*(2), 239–256.

Lorde, A. (2007). *Sister outsider: Essays and speeches by Audre Lorde* (rev ed.). Ten Speed Press.

Lorde, A. (2017). *Your silence will not protect you*. Silver Press.

Leggo, C. (2009). Living love stories: Fissures, fragments, fringes. In M. Prendergast, C. Leggo and P. Sameshima (Eds.) *Poetic inquiry: Vibrant voices in the social sciences*. Sense Publishers. pp. 147–168.

Lyle, E. (2020). Sisterhood and solidarity: Fostering equitable spaces for women in academia. In E. Lyle & S. Mahani (Eds.), *Sister scholars: Untangling issues of identity as women in academe* (pp. 1–10). DIO Press.

Magrini, J. M. (2015). Phenomenology and curriculum implementation: Discerning a living curriculum through the analysis of Ted Aoki's situational praxis. *Journal of Curriculum Studies*, *47*(2), 274–299. https://doi.org/10.1080/00220272.2014.1002113

Maracle, L. (1996). *I am woman: A native perspective on sociology and feminism*. Global Professional Publishing.

Mooney, J. A. (2021a). Moving toward decolonizing and indigenizing curricular and teaching practices in Canadian higher education: An autobiographical narrative exploration. *Learning Landscapes*, *14*(1), 231–247. https://doi.org/10.36510/learnland.v14i1.1045

Mooney, J. A. (2021b). Decolonising academic development practice in Canadian higher education: An autobiographical narrative inquiry into living place-based story [Unpublished manuscript]. Department of Educational Policy Studies, University of Alberta.

Mooney, J. A. (2021c). Settler starting points: A process model for non-indigenous academics decolonising curricular and teaching practices in Canadian higher education [Unpublished manuscript]. Department of Educational Policy Studies, University of Alberta.

Ólafsson, R. F., & Jóhannsdóttir, H. L. (2004). Coping with bullying in the workplace: The effect of gender, age, and type of bullying. *British Journal of Guidance and Counselling*, *32*(3), 319–333.

Oppezzo, M., & Schwartz, D. L. (2014). Giving your ideas some legs: The positive effect of walking on creativity. *Journal of Experimental Psychology: Learning, Memory, and Cognition, 40*(4), 1142–1152. https://doi.org/10.1037/a0036577

Pendergast, M. (2009). Introduction: The phenomena of poetry in research. In M. Prendergast, C. Leggo and P. Sameshima (Eds.) *Poetic inquiry: Vibrant voices in the social sciences.* Sense Publishers. pp. xix–xli.

Pinar, W. (2012). *What is curriculum theory?* (2nd ed.). Routledge.

Regan, P. (2010). *Unsettling the settler within: Indian residential schools, truth telling, and reconciliation in Canada.* UBC Press.

Rundle, D. (2019). Exploring reconciliation in early learning part 1. Denise Rundle, Coordinator of Boroondara Kindergarten. Early Childhood Australia. (13:24). Retrieved from https://www.youtube.com/watch?v=4jZXCLkAmZ4

Sameshima, P., Fidyk, A., James, K., & Leggo, C. (Eds.). (2018). *Poetic inquiry: Enchantment of place.* Vernon Press.

Samnani, A.-K. (2013). The early stages of workplace bullying and how it becomes prolonged: The role of culture in predicting target responses. *Journal of Business Ethics, 113*(1), 119–132.

Selhub, E. M., & Logan, A. C. (2012). *Your brain on nature: The science of nature's influence on your health, happiness, and vitality.* Harper Collins Publishers Ltd.

Simpson, L. B. (2013). *Islands of decolonial love.* Arbeiter Ring Publishing.

Southern, N. L. (2007). Mentoring for transformative learning: The importance of relationship in creating learning communities of care. *Journal of Transformative Education, 5*(4), 329–338. https://doi.org/10.1177/1541344607310576

Smith, L. T. (2012). *Decolonizing methodologies : Research and indigenous peoples* (Second edition). Zed Books.

Tangney, S., Mooney, J. A., & López Vélez, A. L. (2021). Decolonising curricula through collaborative autoethnography: An international study [Unpublished manuscript]. Academic Development. Cardiff Metropolitan University.

Wheatley, M. J. (2007). *Finding our way: Leadership for an uncertain time.* Berrett-Koehler Publishers, Inc.

6 Self-Location as a Disruptive Counternarrative in Teaching and Learning

Kateri Marie Marandola

Positioning Myself within the Research

> We need to revitalize our social and political institutions. The removal of
> internal pain that we individually carry can accomplish this. Healing the
> generational pain and returning us to the healthy basis from which we came
> can return the people to their original state, prior to colonization. It starts
> with an individual that is tired of oppression, colonial domination, and con-
> fusion. It does not mean that we go back to living in longhouses; it means we
> bring the teachings into the present. It means that we start to walk and talk
> and we do that by listening to each other.
>
> (Hill, 2017, p. 9)

The necessity of an educational restructuring has never been more evident
than today. The global pandemic we are facing has shed a distinct light
on the political and social community values we predominantly practise
as our daily norms, without solid cognition of its systemic nature. We are
being confronted with the destructive nature of colonization, witnessing the
nature of our human shortcomings as we try to survive the destruction the
pandemic has had on many aspects of our lives. What impact is this having on our youth, as they watch the political and social turmoil? There is
a significant impact that educational iniquities are having on student well-
being and education. Subranmanian (2021), in the article "The Lost Year in
Education," identifies the significant pressure that the pandemic has put on
education, as the text acknowledges how all children have been impacted
on different levels in terms of their education based on resources and socio-
economic standing. Subranmanian demonstrates that Canadian schools did
provide technology devices as needed, but the ability to do this was based on
school resources. This transition also came with the responsibility to meet
the individual needs of students in a forum unfamiliar to many educators, as
an emergency response in education to the global pandemic. Educators have
come to play a distinct role in the lives of students throughout the continuing pandemic, as they have had to adjust to online learning in order to continue to provide an education, pivot in a moment's time to online learning,

DOI: 10.4324/9781003205296-8

and maintain leadership within their classrooms in order to provide our students with a sense of security.

Hence, the inequities in education have become undeniably evident. Karakose (2021) identifies the pandemic as drawing attention to the socio-economic inequities experienced within the classroom and the home by students as they moved from in-class to remote online learning.

Karakose also draws on the pandemic as being an opportunity to restructure our educational platform to better serve our students. In Canada, our provincial and federal governments have taken steps to support families with funding based on their socio-economic status and to better support the needs of learners from home. However, as Subranmanian (2021) indicates, the disbursement of funds has been poorly monitored. Various levels of government have made efforts to provide for the needs of families and schools in order to close learning gaps. Subranmanian points to the various contributing factors not thoroughly taken into account, such as the needs of learners in particular socio-economic regions, in order to effectively allocate funding. These iniquities have created serious learning gaps for our students combined with the societal structures that impact their lives outside of the school.

As an educator, this pandemic has solidified my belief in cultural awareness, cultural humility, cultural sensitivity, empathy, and compassion in my role with the learner. Our teaching must reflect this approach in order to best support students more equitably. Prior to this pandemic, I had completed my master's of education between September 2016 and December 2019. My research focus was on self-location, an Indigenous research methodology, as a learning tool. I came across this methodology in a course titled "Indigenous Research." I used the methodology to locate myself in learning about Indigenous education and its history in Canada. This methodology called me to identify my previous knowledge and understandings of Indigenous education. The process was intended to help me decolonize my own knowledge and understanding around Indigenous communities and the history of their education as playing a significant role in assimilating and destroying the cultural practices of an entire people. Kovach et al. (2014) identify self-location as a method of connecting ourselves to the research. Self-location is important not only to those who are Indigenous but also to those who are non-Indigenous researchers who wish to position their work within a framework that aligns with Indigenous ways of knowing. This methodology is rooted in the traditional beliefs of Indigenous storytelling. Kovach et al. explain the concept of self-location as a process of decolonizing our thinking by self-locating our current understandings of a particular Indigenous issue, and pursuing research questions from the process of self-location to decolonize our knowledge and understandings of Indigenous culture and traditions.

Self-location is the connection to self and community. Kouri (2021) identifies self-location as a process of decolonizing settler thinking, as well as a method of developing allyship in the process of decolonizing our understandings of Indigenous communities and their history. In this chapter, we will further develop our understanding of the practice of self-location as a counternarrative in education in order to establish the learner in various aspects of the curriculum and as a member of the learning community. Self-location as a mainstream educational approach to learning functions as a counternarrative in the learning process, providing the learner with autonomous development by respecting their knowledge and in turn allowing the learner to share knowledge with peers and teachers to form truths that create community through mutually shared ways of knowing and learning.

This methodology called me to be transparent with myself about what I knew in an effort to be as culturally aware and grow in cultural competence as a descendent of European settlers. The essence of this methodology allowed me as the writer to identify gaps in my knowledge and understanding as I pursued the research of Indigenous education in Canada. I was able to take ownership of my learning through research. This process did so much more for me than help me to uncover the truth in my research. Using self-location as a method to approach my research allowed me to overcome my fear of approaching issues outside of my own experience and come to effectively understand the experience of someone else through empathy. This allowed me to also make cultural connections with Indigenous cultural and traditional practices. The spirituality of Indigenous communities resonates more with me than my own Catholic faith. I came to develop a more personal relationship and bond with my faith, spirituality, and land-based connections. I began to apply this methodology in my teaching practice, as this process became a method of planning and more effective instruction. Self-location became a counternarrative practice in my classroom to advance multicultural education, meeting individual learning needs and centring non-hegemonic curriculum content such as Indigenous history and education in Canada.

The application of self-location as a counternarrative in my teaching practice has become a diagnostic tool over the past five years. As we have entered the pandemic, this practice has given my students the opportunity to learn about who they are as learners. Whether we are approaching Indigenous curriculum content in history and literature, beginning a language unit on poetry in which the students must know themselves as writers and the topics of interest they like to pursue, or beginning a math unit in which they have to identify their previous knowledge, self-location has become a counternarrative for knowing themselves and their peers through the sharing of who they are and where they come from in terms of personal and family histories. This allows them to become individual learners in a learning community in which everyone has their individuality to share with one another. In essence, we decolonize our thinking about each other and the world around us through spiritual connections. Based on this practice of self-location, I am able to gather anecdotal evidence of their knowledge and understanding of themselves, and programme effectively for the learner.

During the 2020–2021 school year, the COVID-19 pandemic was causing students to transition from the classroom to online learning with the rising numbers of positive cases in various regions of Canada and across the globe. In Ontario, our students transitioned on several occasions throughout the school year. Applying self-location in my pedagogy engaged learners in the learning as we explored various topics, allowing them to focus on their own interests and to then move into the curriculum with a strong base of knowing their own learning gaps from this diagnostic approach. Essentially, we were approaching learning from the current knowledge of the learner so they themselves could see their own learning needs through self-location. Specifically, this was very effective in language arts as we approached our unit on poetry. Prior to beginning the unit, I knew my learners well as this was our last language unit for the school year. I knew those who loved to write, and the majority of the 19 students I had, would prefer to avoid it at all costs. As I began to plan the unit, self-location became the foundation for encouraging my writers. I began by self-locating myself as a writer, identifying my favourite authors, why I enjoyed their work, and the topics I was passionate about writing. I then shared my knowledge and experience with poetry as a learner and teacher. I was very honest in how I presented my practices around writing, as the process of self-location allows the writer to make connections to their community. In my experience, if students can identify with you, this makes the room a much safer environment for the learner and is more encouraging to them in their work if they can see your acceptance of your own humanity. Students then created a slideshow presentation following my example in which they also shared their experience and knowledge through the same questions I had created and responded to. Once students presented their knowledge as poets and personal interests, the writing process was simple for them. They knew which topics they would pursue and wrote a poetry anthology as a final assessment of their learning in the unit. The process of self-location allowed my students to gain confidence in their ability and understand that they are capable of effectively and efficiently achieving success as writers of poetry. This process engaged them in learning and demonstrated their academic dedication and achievement beyond their own personal beliefs of themselves and their learning community. What I noted most was their full engagement in the learning process; they were excited to learn and apply their knowledge. This example of the process of applying self-location as a counternarrative to teaching and learning in my poetry unit has been consistent in its application to all areas of the curriculum.

Further, self-location as a counternarrative maintains respect for the autonomy of the learner. In the application of self-location, students delved into their own interests, and in connecting that to the learning they are able to focus on their own personal interests in the development of their writing.

As an educator, this is essential in developing a relationship with the learner to better support their learning needs. They gain confidence from knowing who they are on a more personal level, and to learn about others and subject matter in a fashion that strengthens their sense of belonging in the learning community. I witnessed students sharing their work with each other, helping each other with editing on their own accord, and being interested in their peers without comparing their abilities, strengthening their sense of autonomy and belonging.

Methodology

This research was completed using secondary sources and using self-location as the methodology. Self-location originated as an Indigenous research methodology used to assist the researcher in establishing themselves prior to investigation. Kovach et al. (2014) identify self-location as a settlers' tool to decolonize their beliefs about Indigenous history and culture. Self-location is derived from the Indigenous concept of research; only being credible and intentional coming from one's own personal experience and knowledge. Self-location is the process of the researcher telling their story in connection to their research focus. Drawson et al. (2017) describe the necessity of self-location in the research process of Indigenous culture and history, as the process supports growth in knowledge and understanding of cultural norms and practices. Drawson et al. explain that without the process of self-location, the result is a lack of knowledge of Indigenous culture and history that results in data that is not useful to the Indigenous communities due to generalizations and misconceptions of the people. Hence, self-location as a counternarrative in teaching and learning serves to ameliorate social issues within school communities.

As a first step, I developed my research questions. To develop these research questions, I came to the table with the idea of researching self-location as an educational tool in mainstream education. The development of this concept is a result of the research I have had the opportunity to complete throughout my master's of education journey. I developed the following questions:

1. How does educational scholarship define the term *self-location*?
2. According to research in the area, what range of applications of self-location may be applied to the public school system in Ontario as a counternarrative to teaching and learning?
3. According to educational research findings, how and why might the use of self-location be more supportive of students than a more traditional, teacher-centred approach?

For the purpose of supporting and honouring the Indigenous origin of self-location, I used self-location as my choice of research methodology. In order to tie myself to the data and the concepts within each of the research questions, I established my learning by writing a self-location piece as a portion of my introduction in order to respect the subjective nature of self-location.

The remainder of this chapter will explore the following themes based on the research questions. These themes are

1. Defining self-location.
2. Self-location as a counternarrative to teaching and learning.
3. Supporting student learning through self-location.

Following the aforementioned steps throughout this chapter, I was able to identify specific steps required to implement self-location as a counternarrative in teaching and learning. This teaching practice supported through the data must be experienced by the educator subjectively in order to fully understand the influence of self-location in the learning environment. This is not only beneficial to supporting the decolonization of how we teach and measure success, but also meets the need for decolonizing curriculum and teaching methods regarding Indigenous peoples, and the colonial damage that continues to plague their communities.

Defining Self-Location

Self-location is an Indigenous research methodology suggested as a research approach for settler researchers, as identified by Kovach et al. (2014), for the purpose of approaching research in Indigenous communities. Self-location allows the researcher to establish their position in the research through personal storytelling which identifies the researcher's knowledge related to the area and sets the tone for investigating the research question. Absolon and Willett (2004) identify self-location as integral to establishing our sense of accountability and responsibility to ensure that the research is aligned with the essence of the Indigenous community, in which one may be studying a specific issue. Absolon and Willett, through the presentation of their own experiences as Indigenous researchers, establish that the only voice that can be represented in any research is their own. They further develop the concept of self-location by indicating that self-location is also a path to reclaiming their stories as Indigenous peoples. In practice as an Indigenous or settler researcher, self-location serves to benefit the Indigenous community as it establishes the necessary understandings regarding culture and history, necessary to decolonize the researcher's thinking in the pursuit of improving conditions within the community.

Self-location has acted as a research methodology that allows the Indigenous and settler researcher to bring truth to colonial representations of Indigenous culture and history, empowering Indigenous peoples and communities to reclaim their authentic truth. According to Absolon and Willett (2004), Indigenous research that is approached without the application of self-location by settlers has historically revealed "the patri-archy, paternalism, racism, white supremacy, fear, ignorance and ethno-centrism of their authors than they do about [Indigenous] peoples" (p. 8). Absolon and Willett hold that while not all pre- and post-contact repre-sentations of Indigenous people is misrepresentative of their culture and history without the application of self-location, the cultural ignorance and disregard set the tone for "genocidal policies and practices implemented against [Indigenous] peoples of Canada" (p. 9). Absolon and Willett agree that an analysis of colonization is necessary in order to "decolonize our mind, heart and spirit. Without this critical knowledge, we are operating in a vacuum. Colonization of [Indigenous] peoples could not have been perpetuated and maintained without the role of knowledge extraction and propagation of false consciousness" (p. 9). Absolon and Willett establish the role of self-location in Indigenous research as a form of educational research that reconstructs the representation of Indigenous people through "the crea-tion of written texts that liberate authentic Indigenous knowledges, voices and experiences at individual and collective levels" (p. 10). Self-location allows Indigenous peoples to reclaim their history and culture, leading to the progressive change of policies and practices that previously led to the destruction within their communities.

Additionally, it is held among Indigenous researchers that objectivity cannot function in any form of research that intends to serve a social cause. Absolon and Willett (2004) express that if research is observed through a human lens, neutrality and objectivity do not exist in research. Speaking from the heart and head brings forth the authentic quality of the research. The human element through honest connection is what makes the research and its impact a reality. With this, Absolon and Willett acknowledge that self-location is a tool that benefits any research standpoint that is driven by personal experience. Within self-location, it is essential for the researcher to move to personal experience rather than a broad perspective. This voice that is brought to the research is essential in bringing the transformative element to the research which leads to change. Truth-seeking is how we recover ourselves and the community within our research. Community connection is essential to self-location and makes the research influential in serving the community.

Self-Location as a Counternarrative to Teaching and Learning

The application of Indigenous educational methodologies is a central tool in teaching Indigenous knowledges. These ways of knowing must first be practised by the educator in order to effectively meet the needs of students. Bissell and Korteweg (2016) hold that integrating Indigenous knowledge and teaching approaches is necessary towards promoting intercultural understanding, empathy, and mutual respect. Bissell and Korteweg dis-cuss the use of "Indigenous student-generated digital narratives" that bring to light student "perspectives and voices" as a student learning tool. This form of self-location allows the student to place self in the learning, giving Indigenous learners control of their representation. Bissell and Korteweg express the damning nature of Eurocentric education on Indigenous learners, expressing gaps in learning are determined through standardized assessments among Indigenous students. This process seeks to assimilate learning through settler teaching tools that do not serve Indigenous learners and their needs. To best serve the learner, it is essential to apply learning tools that are culturally aligned with their learning needs.

Similarly, self-location as a counternarrative for teaching and learning among Indigenous and non-Indigenous learners and educators is a holistic approach towards engaging the individual with the larger learning community. Blimkie et al. (2014) define this approach as an "Indigenous philosophical concept of holism," referring to the entity of an individual's intellectual and spiritual realms that form a "whole healthy person." Further, Blimkie et al. identify the impact of self-location on cross-cultural learning, as we all maintain one common goal in our learning working towards "balance and harmony so that no one realm is privileged over another" (p. 50). Here we see self-location as a tool towards holism, allowing each individual to share their location and develop mutual understanding in the process that best supports relationships and community.

Furthermore, land-based education reflects self-location as it places Indigenous knowledge at the centre of learning, an approach to learning that places community and Indigenous experience as key to inheriting knowledge and life skills. Land-based education is an Indigenous learning approach in which the learner investigates connections to the land on which they live, and learn from Elders how to use and live on the land in line with cultural norms and values that serve the greater community. Calderon (2014) brings to attention the work of decolonization through land-based education, as it aims to decolonize the local community in order to understand how colonialism has impacted the community historically and presently to better inform how to move forward. Self-location through land education equips settlers and Indigenous communities to move towards decolonizing the impacts of colonialism, building relationships and community that result in healing and restitution. This approach in mainstream education broadens the scope of restitution, in the process facilitating reciprocal community connections between Indigenous communities, outside agencies, and persons.

Further, literature is a universal tool that in any context has served to educate and develop connections between cultures and communities. Gonzalez et al. (2010) observe the use of literature as a tool that informs our understanding and perspectives about the world around us, having a direct impact on how we view the world. Gonzalez et al. identify these narratives as providing a foundation that directly impacts perceptions and influences how we relate to the land and its people. Gonzalez et al. highlight how children's literature, most notably picture books, can serve non-Indigenous educators in recognizing their preconceived notions gained through colonial knowledge and literature. Gonzalez et al. identify this shift in colonized frames of reference, as the gateway to the decolonization of non-Indigenous education. Gonzalez et al. highlight, as an example of literature as a self-location tool towards decolonization, the connections that can be made between the environmental crisis and its connection with "colonial damage to Indigenous peoples, their traditional rights and lands" (p. 347). Self-location as a counternarrative to teaching and learning, allows educators and students to deconstruct their preconceived notions of the world around them through questions and discussions that are directed by socioculturally relevant and responsive content. Structuring a curriculum around universal topics that are relatable to all people allows for discussions around issues that have affected all cultures throughout history in both relatable and non-relatable ways, surfacing important issues that impact global relationships across cultures.

Supporting Student Learning through Self-Location

Self-location has the potential to serve students through a holistic approach to learning. This research approach serves to educate the self in order to serve the greater community, while developing authentic relationships that are meant to support unity through self-care and knowledge. Self-location as an educational tool serves the student by engaging them in the learning in a fashion that connects them personally to the learning. This is a self-regulation tool, as being connected to the learning involves the learner's authentic knowledge. Anderson et al. (2015) hold that when students are taught self-management, it results in fewer disruptions that often interfere with learning. Self-management is a result of wanting to be present in the learning, which is the result of engagement that can be supported through self-location.

Therein, self-location serves to educate the child as a whole. This approach as an educational tool supports identities who have experienced trauma, presently and historically. Self-location allows the person to ground themselves in who they are and identify gaps through their story, then to proceed with the learning in a manner that is healing and therapeutic. This supports socio-emotional learning in educational contexts. Anderson et al. (2015) explain that children's behaviour in the classroom can be interpreted as defiance or a lack of respect, when in fact the behaviours are often responses to trauma. They further explain that responses to discipline through zero-tolerance policies are ineffective and retriggering for the child. Anderson et al. encourage positive behaviour supports for students and for educators to "reconceptualize their understanding of the causes of these behaviours as physiological reactions to trauma and overwhelming stress" (p. 131). What is emphasized through the approach of self-location as an educational tool for students who have experienced trauma is the importance of the educator to know the child in order to better serve their educational needs. Indigenous communities experienced intergenerational trauma as a result of colonization. Intergenerational trauma refers to the traumatic impact of the colonization of a population throughout several generations. Due to the ongoing nature of the trauma, they continue to be gravely affected as demonstrated through the intersection of social, political, and economic issues.

With a focus on Indigenous intergenerational trauma, the outright disregard for Indigenous cultural practices and norms were blatant as the Canadian government aimed to assimilate Indigenous peoples with colonial beliefs and practices resulting in cultural genocide through the use of residential schools. Carr-Stewart (2006) identifies the Indian Act of 1876 as being the foundation of Indigenous education to this present day, making all educational programmes and services a part of the federal government's policy to assimilate. Specifically, First Nations people were refused involvement in their child's education. Carr-Stewart continues to describe any pursuit of a post-secondary career that resulted in employment would strip First Nations people of their status. He continues by describing First Nations communities as self-governing prior to confederation, and the Indian Act aimed to remove control of First Nations people in the governance of their own communities and this included education. Carr-Stewart highlights the fact that low-level funding attracted teachers that did not have the education or the vocational calling to make the education of Indigenous children successful, which became an ongoing issue in the on- and off-reserve education. The white Paper of 1969 set into motion Indigenous control over Indigenous education. Carr-Stewart (2006) notes that the white paper's in-depth look at the impacts of colonialism on Indigenous communities set into action the document "*Indian Control of Indian Education*: a statement of educational philosophy, values, and future direction for educational jurisdiction" (p. 10). Education had been used as a tool, and was continuing to be used, to assimilate Indigenous peoples into settler culture. The question becomes, how do we repair the damage and create a better educational system to support Indigenous students?

Dénommé-Welch and Montero (2014) identify three factors that impede the success of Indigenous control over Indigenous education: lack of cultural knowledge amongst educators, lack of proper representation of Indigenous history and culture in the curriculum, and the absence or poor delivery of Indigenous educational approaches to meet the needs of the Indigenous learner. Dénommé-Welch and Montero (2014) describe the process of colonization as one that has suppressed Indigenous knowledge systems, and contributed to low levels of educational achievement, as well as a wealth of social issues such as high rates of suicide, incarceration, unemployment, and family dysfunction. This has its roots in intergenerational trauma and the perpetuation of colonial logic and its deficit thinking. They continue to make the connection that the lack of awareness among educators of

Indigenous history and culture is also a result of colonization, claiming that the "cloud of colonization is sustained in teacher education programs because Indigenous education and Indigenous knowledge systems continue to be marginalized" (p. 138). There is a distinct call for teacher education around Indigenous history and culture in Canada. This is important to better service Indigenous peoples through acquiring teaching/learning approaches that reflect Indigenous knowledge to tell truths masked by colonial influence. Dénommé-Welch and Montero explain that the challenge for most educators is knowing how to engage with the Indigenous content of the curriculum in a meaningful way as a result of their lack of cultural awareness. Dénommé-Welch and Montero discuss the education of preservice teachers and the necessity for them to understand how the curriculum "oppresses and undermines" Indigenous peoples (p. 148); this is suggesting that storytelling, as a self-location educational approach, is a necessary collaborative effort towards decolonization, as Elders share the history and culture to inform the misconceptions of a colonial education system.

In addition to misconceptions presented in the curriculum that falsely and inadequately represent Indigenous peoples, many social issues are attributed to colonial influences. Desai (2016), from the perspective of the "Filipina/o American" experience of colonization, emphasizes the necessity of acknowledging and acting on the impacts of colonialism to effectively address traumas that plague communities today. Education offers a unique opportunity to support new learning approaches that answer to the urgency of decolonizing the curriculum, as well as beliefs and practices that are detrimental to Indigenous peoples. Educators play a central role in this development, which requires them to decolonize their own beliefs and practices involving Indigenous peoples. Halagao (2004) draws attention to the fact that our perspectives are rooted in our lived experiences which are often unexamined. He concludes that if teachers want to provide equitable and meaningful learning opportunities for all learners, they "need to understand how students experience particular curricula that challenge their prior knowledge, ethnic identities, and relationships with others" (p. 462). This is a call for a complete revamping of how we teach and learn in educational spaces. Our education system impacts all students and its stakeholders, as it is strongly influenced by colonial beliefs and practices that maintain and reflect a system that is detrimental to the development of self and, in turn, community. This insight points us in the direction of finding commonality among our students and educators to understand what has happened in our Canadian history within and outside education, so that we may heal from the colonial experience as a nation. This is the purpose of self-location; discovering our own story and that of our peers, so that we can empathize and live as allies with a strong sense of self and our role in the greater community. Tanya Talaga (2017) describes the dangers of not knowing the Indigenous history of Canada with a focus on Northern Ontario communities in her book *Seven Fallen Feathers: Racism, Death, and Hard Truths in a Northern*

City. Through her cultural practice of storytelling, Talaga points us to the ongoing lived trauma of Indigenous communities in Northern Ontario as continued contributors to intergenerational trauma created largely by the residential school experience. The poor living conditions on reserves and systemic racism continue to impact these communities and will take generations to heal. Talaga points to the importance of educating our children about our history and understanding of Indigenous culture and traditional practices to become allies of decolonization. Self-location as an educational practice supports this development as students develop a strong sense of self and community by making connections through the practice of empathy.

Additionally, learning within Indigenous communities is a cultural practice that involves oral traditions. There is a great emphasis on learning through relationships and community building. Lambe (2003) discusses various Indigenous communities and their oral traditions, noting that teaching and learning within these communities is based on relationship building with an individual; the educator being the mentor who respects the autonomy of the learner by listening and making suggestions to guide their learning, in which they have options as opposed to making the suggestions an obligation, allowing the learner to "be free to regard, disregard, or continue to reflect, depending on how the person feels" (p. 309). Lambe holds that the nature of this form of education has a profound effect due to its personal nature, where learning is nurtured through personal connection but "not forced or dictated. One is never told what to learn or how one should learn it. Learning is entirely dependent on the willingness of the elder and mentor and the person's respect, motivation, interests and gifts" (p. 309). Mainstream educational practices are regulated with a great emphasis on content, standards of achievement, and measures of success. It embodies a standardized way of learning that, if not met, indicates a discrepancy in the learner's ability to learn. Although I have witnessed teaching approaches come into practice that are similar in nature, they continue to maintain a universal goal of meeting a specific standardized curriculum that defines a successful learner. There appears to be little regard for the autonomy of the learner even though we have come to recognize the necessity. Subsequently, self-location offers an element in mainstream education that respects the learner's personal experience, knowledge base, and interests built on the foundation of establishing an understanding of the self, followed by relationship building and community connections. Indigenous knowledge base reflected in self-location brings to the forefront the importance of personal development and mobilization to challenge systemic injustices.

Conclusion

Self-location as an educational tool provides an exploration of self in connection to resources to establish and affirm one's own knowledge in partnership with peers, others, and the larger community. Establishing the structure of self-location as an educational tool serves the holistic development of students by supporting their mind, body, spirit, and community. Wisselink (2019) in "An Indigenous Pedagogy for Colonization" describes the role of self-location as making the area of focus an embodied journey as well as an approach that welcomes a more "holistic" and "soulful way of knowing." Although self-location was originally established and is identified as an Indigenous research methodology, through these findings we have come to see its significance as having an essential role in education. Self-location has the potential to serve the mainstream learning community in a variety of ways that facilitate learning in subject matters that allows the child to identify their own understandings in all areas to establish their own values and make connections to their social worlds. Once self-knowledge and understandings are established, this opens the forum for the learner to investigate their beliefs through a variety of methods that reflect relationship building with tools to deconstruct and unlearn beliefs of Indigenous history and culture, and, in turn, service the Indigenous community as truths are established among the settler culture regarding their colonial experience.

Self-location has the potential to positively impact students' ability to connect to the learning, and with this connection comes self-regulation within the learning environment. As mental health has become increasingly concerning among our youth, self-location serves to promote healing from trauma by engaging pain and suffering as a pedagogy. The significant intergenerational trauma that continues to plague Indigenous communities requires restitution that may be facilitated through self-location. As a result, it is recommended that educators first decolonize their own thinking with regard to settler approaches to education and their understanding of Indigenous communities in terms of culture and colonial impact. Integrating the experience of self-location into teacher education allows teachers to be prepared with the knowledge to effectively service their students in a manner that prepares them for the world around them, while decolonizing their thinking and understandings regarding Indigenous peoples. We must change how we teach and what we teach, as we cannot deny how education impacts societal outcomes.

References

Absolon, K., & Willett, C. (2004). Aboriginal research: Berry picking and hunting in the 21st century. *First Peoples Child and Family Review*, 1(1), 5–17.

Anderson, E. M., Blitz, L. V., & Saastamoinen, M. (2015). Exploring a school-university model for professional development with classroom staff: Teaching trauma-informed approaches. *School Community Journal*, 25(2), 113–134.

Bissell, A., & Korteweg, L. (2016). Digital narratives as a means of shifting settler-teacher horizons toward reconciliation. *Canadian Journal of Education*, 9(3), 1–25.

Blimkie, M., Vetter, D., & Haig-Brown, C. (2014). Shifting perspectives and practices: Teacher candidates' experiences of an aboriginal infusion in mainstream teacher education. *Brock Education: A Journal of Educational Research and Practice, 23*(2), 47–66.

Calderon, D. (2014). Speaking back to manifest destinies: A land education-based approach to critical curriculum inquiry. *Environmental Education Research, 20*(1), 24–36.

Carr-Stewart, S. (2006). The changing educational governance of first nations schools in Canada: Towards local and education equity. *Management in Education, 20*(5), 6–12.

Dénommé-Welch, S., & Montero, M. K. (2014). De/Colonizing preservice teacher education: Theatre of the academic absurd. *Journal of Language and Literacy Education, 10*(1), 136–165.

Desai, M. (2016). Critical "Kapwa": Possibilities of collective healing from colonial trauma. *Educational Perspectives, 48*(1–2), 34–40.

Drawson, A., Toombs, E., & Mushquash, C. (2017). Indigenous research methods: A systemic review. *The International Indigenous Policy Journal, 8*(2). Retrieved from https://www.proquest.com/openview/2eae1e704af8223671bd4c9c6bce7cb1/1?pq-origsite=gscholar&cbl=1996357

Gonzalez, I., Guillet, J., & Korteweg, L. (2010). The stories are the people of the land: Three educators respond to environmental teachings in indigenous children's literature. *Environmental Education Research, 16*(3–4), 331–350.

Halagao, P. E. (2004). Holding up the mirror: The complexity of seeing your ethnic self in history. *Theory and Research in Social Education, 32*(4), 459–483.

Hill, B. H. (2017). *Shaking the tattle: Healing the trauma of colonization.* CreateSpace Independent Publishing Platform.

Karakose, T. (2021). Emergency remote teaching due to COVID-19 pandemic and potential risks for socioeconomically disadvantaged students in higher education. *Educational Process: International Journal, 10*(3), 53–62.

Kouri, S. (2021). Settler education: Acknowledgement, self-location, and settler ethics in teaching and learning. *International Journal of Child, Youth and Family Studies, 11*(3), 56–79.

Kovach, M., Carriere, J., Barrett, M. J., Montgomery, H., & Gilles, C. (2014). Stories of diverse identity locations in indigenous research. In C. Campbell, H. Montgomery, & H. Ritenburg (Guest Eds.), *Special edition of the international review of qualitative research: Indigenous inquiries, 6*(4), 487–509.

Lambe, J. (2003). Indigenous education, mainstream education, and native studies: Some considerations when incorporating indigenous pedagogy into native studies. *American Indian Quarterly, 27*(1/2), 308–324.

Subranmanian, S. (2021, June). The lost year in education. *MacLean's.* Retrieved from https://www.macleans.ca/longforms/covid-19-pandemic-disrupted-schooling-impact/

Talaga, T. (2017). *Seven fallen feathers: Racism, death, and truths in a northern city.* House of Anansi Press Inc.

Wisselink, K. (2019, February 14). *An Indigenous pedagogy for decolonization.* Athabasca University Press. Retrieved from https://www.aupress.ca/blog/2019/02/14/decolonization/

7 Engaging in Ethical Discourse

An Autoethnography of a Black Student's Journey to Self-Identity

Alicia Noreiga

I closed my eyes and counted to five in a futile attempt to hold back tears as I read aloud the remarks posted on the online forum. I read my former professor's comment from the audience's questions and remarks section during the airing of an online student-led panel discussion. The discussion formed part of a New Brunswick university's series of activities in its third year of recognizing Black History Month. The panellists comprised four Black students enrolled at the university. I, also a university student, was privileged to serve as the event's co-organizer and session moderator. The silence that preceded me reading the professor's greetings, accompanied by the look of pain in all panellists' eyes, signified the consolidated feelings of despair and loss resulting from the only Black professor accepting a university position in a more diverse province. Albeit I can only assume the professor's justification for leaving, I posit that being the lone Black faculty member in a predominantly white institution, and further exacerbated by her femininity, can be challenging. In a study to explore the experiences of racialized and Indigenous faculty at Canadian universities, Mohamed and Beagan (2019) concluded that participants experienced everyday racism and colonialism embedded in their university cultures, which the participants found to be often exhausting to deal with. The authors also found that university initiatives aimed at facilitating diversity often fall short of fostering equity. In an earlier study involving 89 racialized faculty at 10 Canadian universities, Henry and Tator (2012) found racism embedded in the institutions' structures, as many racialized faculty, especially Black women, expressed feelings of loneliness and alienation within their universities.

With the professor's departure, already scarce mentorship became non-existent. The absence of Black staff to serve as mentors and counsel to the university's small percentage of Black students was one of the several issues the Black student panellists discussed as they disclosed experiences and opinions regarding anti-Black racism, articulated from the vantage points of Black[1] students. Some of Canada's citizens, especially those belonging to the dominant white population, may view this unveiling of experiences with racism with acrimony, as our revelations jeopardized the façade that Canada is an unblemished representation of equity and human rights (Gulliver, 2018;

DOI: 10.4324/9781003205296-9

Mensah, 2010). The misguided belief that racism and racial segregation is not a Canadian issue masks the realities that African Canadians face daily (Reynolds, 2016). My ability to organize and moderate this event created a space for added discourse on Black issues in Canada's education and served as an empowering tool towards my growing Black activism.

In this chapter, I present an autoethnographic account of my experiences as a Black international woman attending a New Brunswick university. I examine the complexities of my identity as I grappled with becoming Black, then being Black (see also Noreiga, 2020). Forced into accepting a racial label – Black – then embracing the significance and role of a Black woman in higher education, I ask, How has racism in Canada influenced my understanding of who I am and my role in higher education? To answer this question, I first reflect on my experiences with racism in my home country, Trinidad and Tobago. I next explore my experiences with racism in Canada and the ways my new circumstances shaped my identity and my understanding of what it means to be Black in New Brunswick. Further, I share ways I capitalized on my newly founded identity as an empowering tool to support activism and create safer spaces for fellow students. Finally, I recount one experience moderating a discussion with four Black university students and the ways I capitalized on the opportunity to provide *ethical facilitation* (Brown & Danaher, 2017; Graham, Powell, & Truscott, 2016) to create a *safer space* (hooks, 1994; The Roestone Collective, 2014) for Black students.

African Canadian Feminist Thought

Nestled within the African Canadian feminist lens, my beliefs support Wane et al.'s (2002) opinion that there needs to be a unique theoretical framework for Black women and, more so, Black women in Canada. Literature, grounded on feminist theories, is often written, pioneered, and reflective of white women's lives. Feminist theory frequently excludes the juxtaposing experiences that race creates. Black women experience multiple oppressions, including being women and being Black (hooks, 1981; Lorde, 2019). Already subjected to racial subordination, Black women's gender also compounds their already oppressed situation. Thus, the birth of Black feminist thought fills the void left in feminist research. Wane (2002) defines Black feminist thought as

> a theoretical tool meant to elucidate and analyze the historical, social, cultural, and economic relationships of women of African descent to develop a liberatory praxis. It is a paradigm grounded in the historical and contemporary experiences of Black women as mothers, activists, academics, and community leaders. (p. 38)

Black American women, such as bell hooks and Patricia Hill Collins, significantly shaped Black feminism. Although their work and philosophies created fundamental understandings of feminist theories and Black women's experiences, I concur with Wane et al. (2002) that African American feminist thought does not always correlate directly and fully to African Canadian experiences. Racism is experienced differently for Black women in Canada and Black women in America. In some cases, the overt forms of racism women experience in the United States may exist in more subtle forms in Canada. I go further to declare that racism looks differently for Black women residing in different parts of Canada due to each province's differing demographics and culture that impact the presence and experience of various minority groups. There is, therefore, a need for fundamental theorizing to coalesce the unique experiences of Black women living in Canada. African Canadian feminist theories place Black Canadian women at the nexus of analysis and allow their diverse voices to become unified empowering tools in opposing racism and white dominance from a Canadian perspective.

Methodological Framing

In this chapter, I employ autoethnography as the overarching methodological approach as a form of resistance as I speak back against anti-Black racism in Canada. Autoethnography is a qualitative research methodology that places the *self* at the nexus of the phenomenon under investigation by stimulating critical self-reflection of first-hand experiences with the phenomenon (Rambo & Ellis, 2020; Singleton, 2020). Autoethnography allows socially marginalized voices to enter academic discourse (Marx, Pennington, & Chang, 2017) and creates opportunities for persons to disseminate their first-hand accounts of ways power and privilege played out in their personal lives. Through autoethnography, Black scholars have become active participants in educating marginalized and dominant groups about racist actions, challenging the status quo of normalizing systemic racism, and transforming racist practices (examples include Mekonen, 2021; Wane et al., 2002)

Black feminist autoethnography considers the complexities and multilayered experiences of Black women (see Henry, 2015; Hernandez, Ngunjiri, & Chang, 2015; Hill, Callier, & Waters, 2019; McCarthy, 2006, 2014; Mogadime, 2002; Osei, 2019). Key to Black feminism is the empowerment of Black women through their voices that were previously silenced in traditional feminist theory (hooks, 1981). Adding to these crucial discourses, I present my narrative, as a point of Black Canadian feminist discourse, on the ways racism is a reality for Black international students, and call on my fellow Black women to empower themselves by becoming proactive contributors in unveiling concealed systemic racism, form solidarities, and amplify their voices in academia.

From Majority

I am Black, yet in Trinidad and Tobago, I never needed to declare my racial identity. The most southerly Caribbean island, Trinidad and Tobago's population comprises 98% dark-coloured descendants, of which 40% are of African heritage, 40% Indian heritage, and 18% are considered to be mixed. Yet, the country's 0.6% white population is perceived to be the most powerful ethnic group – a legacy of colonialism. Brand (2001), a Trinidadian writer who migrated to Canada, described Trinidad and Tobago as a country where citizens do not remember Africa, yet it remains in the identity of who they are. I often take my African heritage for granted, as most citizens are Black and people of colour. The African Diaspora, during slavery, and the Indian diaspora, after slavery, along with the lesser presence of Indigenous, Spanish, British, French, Chinese, and Lebanese inhabitants, created the country's dominant African, Indian, and mixed race. The intermixing of races – common among Caribbean islands –resulted in my mosaic racial identity: an ancestral lineage from continental Africa, Europe, and Indigenous South America. With Jim Crow laws never overtly implemented following the abolition of slavery, many Trinidadians perceived racism, white dominance, and Black segregation as issues present in other countries. My *Caribbean privilege* – a shield from overt anti-Black racism and white dominance – allowed me to grow up in a world where my race is normalized and gender segregation is more prominent than racial segregation. I grew up seeing representations of my race in leadership and mentorship positions, such as Black prime ministers, presidents, judges, businesspersons, and other affluent members of society. Although I acknowledged my ancestors' dehumanization by whites who have since relinquished control of our citizenry and migrated to their home countries, I feel pride in belonging to a country where "every creed and race find an equal place" (national anthem of Trinidad and Tobago). Or do they?

Trinidad and Tobago has strategically concealed the apparent racism that affords dominant entitlement to the 0.6% white citizenry. Residing in the more affluent areas within the country and attending the more prestigious schools, Trinidadian whites have historically benefited from the colonialist systems that advantaged persons of lighter hues. Primarily persons of Lebanese heritage, the country's local whites migrated to Trinidad to substitute African slaves following the abolition of slavery, as former slaves refused employment at the plantations where they endured inhumane treatment. Soon after migrating to the country, these lighter-skinned workers realized that their complexion created employment opportunities which other immigrant workers from countries such as China and India, along with the Black locals, could not access. For instance, during the early twentieth century, most of the country's banks were Canadian-owned (Hébert, 2016). At these banks, local whites found employment opportunities that Black people could not, which resulted in the country's whites acquiring higher income to purchase land, houses, and start businesses (Cudjoe, 2017; Hébert, 2016). The 1970 Black Power Revolution in Trinidad and Tobago – as an act of protest against racism in Canada – dismantled many of these overt racial structures. In 1969 several university students in Trinidad took to the streets in the country's capital in support of Trinidadians facing trial in Canada due to their 1968 acts of protest towards blatant forms of racism that West Indian students endured at Montreal's Sir George University. This led to the birth of the Black Power revolution in Trinidad. As Hébert expressed, "Young Trinidadians saw Black Power as a challenge to the fact that political independence [in Trinidad and Tobago] had not changed an economic system in which skin color still dictated a person's employment opportunities." Reacting to these conditions and embracing racial consciousness, the country's post-independence generation engaged in activism that initiated eventual awareness and action against Black suppression. However, local whites had already experienced significant upward economic mobility and, thus, secured their place as the country's dominant racial economic group. Today, their small white population allows them to strategically downplay their presence as the country's dominant society. In his 2017 award-winning CNN series *Parts Unknown*, Anthony Bourdain produced an episode on Trinidad and Tobago during which he interviewed Mario Sabga-Aboud, a member of the 0.6% white citizenry. In this interview Sabga-Aboud expressed his opinion that the white population was the most powerful ethnic group in the country (Sweet, 2017). Local activists such as Cudjoe (2017) deemed Sabga-Aboud's declaration a reminder of the country's dominance by an elite minority group which continues to enjoy advantages in terms of urbanization, access to education, and public sector employment. Hundreds of millions of dollars in government contracts are awarded to local white elites on a yearly basis (Cudjoe, 2017), whereas other groups are not offered the same financial opportunity. In a subsequent television interview, Gary Aboud responded to public condemnation of Sabga-Aboud's statements (IS T&T, 2017). Aboud (a member of the white community) expressed shock by citizens' resentment and claimed that Bourdain's story was edited with the intention of profiling and creating a misconception of arrogance among his community. He voiced the opinion that cliques, social division, and inequity are normal. In concert with Freire's (2002) description of dominant groups' attempts to justify and shield their domination, Aboud proclaimed that his group worked hard and was therefore entitled to their earnings and social lifestyle, and rebuked any blame for their success. I do not refute the notion that this dominant group worked hard for its achievements. However, I posit that members need to acknowledge their privilege, which made their journey to success easier as opposed to the experiences of marginalized groups.

Amidst the colonialist regime that maintains the white race's historical dominance over Black people, Trinidad and Tobago's Black citizens longer encounter explicit suppression as they continue to experience upward education and economic mobility. The notion that persons are less likely to be successful because they are Black is not a local reality, but instead accompanies the realism that all whites are likely to be successful because they are white. As I left Trinidad destined for better education opportunities in

Canada, I bore the identity of a woman who has overcome many challenges such as growing up in a small rural impoverished village and gender inequities as I reflect on my years as one of the first four female lifeguards in Trinidad. Entering a male-dominated work environment, we were met with macro- and microaggressions. We were destined to prove ourselves worthy amidst a lack of female facilities and both male colleagues and beach-goers rejecting our positions as they openly expressed opinions that females were unfit to perform rescues. We demanded respect and, through our performance, proved that women were equally effective in performing life-saving duties. Our resilience set a precedent that has now resulted in over a dozen female lifeguards employed at beaches throughout the country. As I began my new chapter as a Canadian resident, the resilience that steered me through local adversities remained with me as I set on a pathway to anticipated professional success.

To Minority

Arriving in New Brunswick, I was unprepared for my newly acquired existence as a member of a minority race. I posit that Canada's education system does little to accommodate the diverse origins of its international students. Although authors such as Dionne Brand and Frances Henry provided vital foundational contributions to the narrative discourse describing education in Canada from Caribbean residents' standpoints, there is a paucity of research that explores Black Caribbean students' experiences as they attend universities in Atlantic Canada (exceptions include Noreiga & Justin, 2021). Noreiga and Justin (2021) explored the ways their Blackness and international status intersected to exacerbate their feelings of isolation both on and off campus. The authors cited culture shock, language barriers, feelings of isolation and loneliness, homesickness, financial constraints, social identity crisis, racism, and an acute awareness of their skin colour as adversities they endured while adjusting and functioning to meet their academic demands. Noreiga and Justin also explored the ways they were able to overcome perpetual obstacles to become advocates and pioneer transformation while successfully completing their post-secondary education objectives. Thus, moving from a country where Black people held a majority racial composition to a country where Black residents are a minority, disadvantaged population was a daunting phenomenon for me. Being a victim of racism and racial segregation threatened all previous assumptions regarding my life and identity.

Whether we grew up in the Caribbean, North America, Britain, or Africa, we have been educated from a colonialist perspective which has taught us to either disregard or disrespect non-whites (Mathienson, 2002). Systemic racism is a normative aspect of Canada's university culture (Henry, 2015). I experienced the reality of Mathienson's statements (2002) as I leverage my life as a Black student in a white institution, void of any recognition or accommodation for Black people and people of colour. The total erasure of Black history perpetuated a perception that Black Canadians were either non-existent in the development or only arrived in Canada through recent migration from the Caribbean and Africa. Nowhere within my university experience did I see my race reflected and recognized as integral to the province's development. Void of Black professors, non-janitorial staff, and courses that focused specifically on Black histories or anti-racism, I was left with the impression that the university perceived communities of colour as insignificant.

Mogadime (2002) maintained that Canada's higher education institutions pose particular challenges to Black women and other women of colour who are graduate students and faculty. Via her autoethnographic account, Mogadime described the challenges Black graduate students endure as they grapple with finding academic socialization and professional development opportunities. As I struggled to understand my new experiences, my need for social interaction and mentorship became obvious. The dearth of Black faculty staff prevented Black students from forming social attachments with other Black academics. There was little or no opportunity to have professional or personal discussions with Black professors or colleagues. Instead, the feelings of isolation and detachment from the university and my faculty engulfed me (Noreiga, 2020). I needed a confidant, someone to serve as a counsellor. I longed for someone that could relate to my complicated situation and offer reassuring words of comfort and advice.

In this *great white North* (Baldwin, Cammeron, & Kobayashi, 2012), Canadians expect Black international students to assimilate into the Canadian ethos. I felt pressured to abandon my identity, culture, and lifestyle, and replace it with the dominant groups' expected behaviours. After a couple of weeks in New Brunswick, I recall my sheer jubilation on seeing a beautiful bodice on the *sales* rack at a department store. I was elated that I could purchase such a beautiful item that would cost significantly higher back home. The following day, shame replaced my pride when I entered my classroom, and my professor looked at me in amazement and remarked, "What a bright shirt!" I realized that my cultural background, which influenced my Caribbean fashion sense, was now considered unsuitable. I was now not only a Black woman, but I was also a Black woman who dresses inappropriately. My blouse now lays in a suitcase destined to be worn on my next visit to Trinidad, where I can parade in my bright colours without a feeling of *otherness*.

The perception that all Black people are homogeneous disregards the differences among the 2% Black New Brunswickers. Black Canadians are heterogeneous (Wane et al., 2002). Their experience with racism is the primary factor that brings them together. Just as Black people migrating to Canada from African countries share diverse cultures, languages, and practices, so are Canadian-born and Black people from the Caribbean. In 2019, two white women invited me to a Caribbean carnival celebration in one of

New Brunswick's cities. Not realizing that I was a Trinidadian, they promised that the event would be similar to Trinidad's carnival. Having realistic expectations, I did not anticipate a celebration comparable to Trinidad's, but I expected a simplified version of Ontario's Caribana and was, thus, anxious to hear calypso and soca[2] and see costumes to rejuvenate my connection to home. To my utter disappointment, Trinidad carnival's music did not form part of the event's entertainment. Instead, dancers in their costumes paraded to African music that had little resemblance to the Caribbean carnival's birthplace. The disregard for Black diversity resulted in the event's organizers, whom I presume were white, considering any Black person knowledgeable about Caribbean carnival and cultures. To further exacerbate my disappointment, I was confident that the organizers, nor anyone present, knew that Trinidad's carnival was a celebration of Black liberation from slavery where the finally freed slaves mocked the slave owners' dress as they paraded the streets. From those portrayals emerged the artistry that now signifies Trinidad, and by extension, Caribbean carnival. I commend the organizer's efforts to include diversity in the province's cultural recognitions, but I posit that more dedication must be given to researching the heterogeneity of Black cultures to ensure that Black people do not witness their unique identities and cultures being demeaned.

Becoming Black

Freire (2002) positioned knowledge as the impetus to liberation. He implored persons experiencing oppression to educate themselves and their oppressors if they desire positive transformation. Being a Black female outsider in a white dominant province can be intimidating, to say the least. However, as my new racialized reality set in, I knew that being Black meant more than merely understanding the disadvantages that come with my label. I now needed to find my voice and embrace my power as an emerging Black female scholar. I longed to seek Black connections, which I was confident was present in New Brunswick. My journey to unveiling Black presence in New Brunswick began with reading *Viola Desmond's Canada*, where I was astounded to learn of Atlantic Canada's rich Black history that dated back over 250 years. With a new appetite for knowledge to seal my Black identity, I perused books such as *Racial Discrimination in Canada, Colour-Coded: A Legal History of Racism in Canada, Black Canadians, The Blacks in New Brunswick*, and *The Book of Negros*. I was surprised that the province's policymakers successfully suppressed such essential aspects of the province's history from education forums and discourses. I was equally surprised to learn of the substantial number of West Indians, including Trinidadians, that migrated to the province between 1900 and 1960 (Reynolds, 2016) and Atlantic Canada's role in Black oppression in areas such as Africville, Nova Scotia, where Black settlements were dismantled by oppressive white settlers (Backhouse, 1999).

Black people always played an integral role in New Brunswick's develop-ment. Spray (1972) traced Black people's presence in New Brunswick before the province's establishment. Then in 1783, over 3,000 free Black loyalists settled in Nova Scotia and New Brunswick. Although treated poorly and inferior to whites, from then onwards, Black people played integral roles in the province's development. Through Black people's resilience, several influ-ential Black New Brunswickers emerged. These Black New Brunswickers are not recognized alongside the influential New Brunswickers observed in edu-cation forums. I learned of Black New Brunswickers such as Willie O'Ree, Canada's first Black NFL player; Abraham Beverley Walker, Canada's first Afro-Canadian lawyer; Arthur St. George Richardson, the first Black person to attend the University of New Brunswick; and Mary Matilda Winslow, the first Black woman to attend the University of New Brunswick. I opt to conclude my list here as my long record of unearthed influential Black New Brunswickers, past and present, is sufficient to earn a paper of its own.

Learning of the several ways Black New Brunswickers contributed to the province's growth also meant learning of the hidden realities of his-torical Black oppression and the dehumanizing of Black residents perpe-trated by the province's whites. Spray (1972), Walker (1985), and Reynolds (2016) comprehensively researched slavery in the province. The scholars revealed histories of unjust treatment and broken promises Black loyalists received when they arrived at the province with their fellow white loyalists. Despite a promise for equal resources, Black New Brunswickers were given smaller plots of land in far less suitable areas for farming. Their inadequate resources created devastating living conditions, and eventually, the prov-ince's Black residents resorted to working for whites on their prime plots of land to evade poverty and death. In 1792, intentional Black suppression pushed many Black Nova Scotians and New Brunswickers to migrate to Sierra Leone. Disregarding the apparent ill-treatment aimed towards the province's Black population, whites placed sole blame on Black residents' unwillingness to sacrifice and inability to handle the responsibility of free-dom as the reasons for their underdevelopment (Mensah, 2010; Spray, 1972). Learning of Black peoples' contributions also meant learning of the province's 17 active Ku Klux Klan Lodges – *Klaverns* – between 1925 and 1930, where members participated in cross-burnings in most major cities (Backhouse, 1999; Reynolds, 2016). It also meant learning of the ways Black New Brunswickers were excluded and segregated in the province's schools and churches (Spray, 1972).

By hiding Black New Brunswickers' existence from education forms, the province's policymakers are influential in perpetuating the lie that stimu-lates the naïve impression that slavery never existed in Canada. Many believe the country's sole role in Black racism was as a haven for Black people via the underground railroad. These notions exclude the reality that the underground railroad led to freedom from slavery but did not lead to equity, equality, and full participation in Canadian life, and one of the rare instances where conservatives and liberals joined in solidarity was in their quest to make immigration racially restrictive by preventing Black people from coming to Canada (Mensah, 2010; Walker, 1985). My newly founded knowledge goes against the Canadian narrative that Canada is void of a history of racial oppression and inferiorization. My experiences and knowledge gained from recently published literature that African Canadians authored, revealed a still pronounced presence of racial inequities.

Finding My Voice

Having acquired knowledge of Black history and racism in Canada, along with my personal experiences with racism, I found it necessary to use my knowledge as an empowering tool to support other Black New Brunswickers and myself in growing understandings of Black identities. I did not desire to allow my pain and suffering to go unnoticed or prevent me from reaching out to others who may be experiencing the same. I wanted to work towards diverting the trajectory of silenced Black voices in academic spaces. I understood dialogue as a means of transformation (Freire, 2002; hooks, 1994). I believed engaging in ethical discourse with both oppressors and persons experiencing oppression would be one way of counteracting concealed racial issues and pioneering social justice. I, thus, began seeking ways to amplify my voice as a Black international woman and student. My first initiative involved authoring a newspaper article that I published in one of the province's newspapers. In the article, I shared my experiences as a Black international student and the feelings of segregation and identity conflicts Black international students face (Noreiga, 2020). Second, In December 2019–January 2020, I held a series of cellphilm (cellphone + filmmaking) workshops for Black students attending two of New Brunswick's universities. Cellphilm is a contemporary participatory research approach whereby participants use their smart devices to create and disseminate short videos about social justice and equity issues (MacEntee, Burkholder, & Schwab-Cartas, 2016). During these workshops, participants produced short videos to effectively stimulate discussions and raise awareness of racial challenges both local and international Black students experience. Following the workshops, I used my position as an emerging Black scholar and active member of several university committees to disseminate participants' cellphilms in several academic and non-academic forums (see Noreiga, in press).

Facilitating Ethical Discourse

My most recent initiative involved planning and moderating a panel discussion with students attending one of New Brunswick's universities. Following Freire's (2002) guidelines, I believe that it is the duty of persons experiencing oppression to discuss their oppressive states. As such, I felt it necessary for the university's Black students to discuss their experiences and vocalize their feelings in a manner that empowers and stimulates activism. It is difficult and at times harmful for Black students to talk about racism. I was aware of the negative drawbacks associated with Black activism. Kelley (2018) identified ways Black students experienced adverse consequences for their activism, such as victimization, further isolation, and occurrences whereby the dominant student community denounce Black international students' critiques and accuse them of being unappreciative of the opportunity for better education. Thus, it was my duty to create a safer space for my Black panellists. Safe spaces are institutional, systemic creations that ensure marginalized groups are free from violence and harassment (King, 2020; The Roestone Collective, 2014). In *Teaching to Transgress*, hooks (1994) endorsed the importance of safe environments for Black students and other marginalized groups where they can speak freely, form collective strength, and generate resilience strategies without fear of victimization. These safe spaces must be present throughout the institution, thus becoming part of the school's ethos.

To create a safer space for panellists, I engaged everyone throughout the process. I involved all panellists in planning the event. I sought their feedback in determining the questions and the parameters of the discussion. We met on two occasions to determine the theme and topics that students felt safe and comfortable enough to discuss. I then invited each participant to submit one question they would like to explicitly address during the event. By allowing panellists the autonomy to compose their primary questions, the students could speak of issues that were dear to them. After all participants submitted their questions, I made the interview protocol available to all panellists days before the event to allow them the opportunity to plan their responses and to suggest any question that they prefer not to address or prefer addressing. This action was important to me as I felt it integral to allow the space for participants to tell their stories in the way they deem necessary.

I was constantly cognizant that I needed to be an ethical facilitator if I were to effectively capitalize on the panel discussion as a medium of empowerment and activism. Ethical facilitation entails creating an environment of trust and solidarity with a genuine desire to empower persons to be active participants in positively transforming their lives (Brown & Danaher, 2017; Graham, Powell, & Truscott, 2016). To achieve this type of facilitation, I first needed to generate avenues to foster mutual trust and panellists' comfort in viewing me as a comrade with similar experiences. hooks (1994) postulated that persons facilitating safe and ethical discourse must be willing to share confessional narratives. By sharing my stories, I became less of a silent interrogator and more a comrade in solidarity with all other students. Thus, it was important that, throughout the event, I, too, shared my experiences as a Black international student. During the discussion, I admitted my internal conflicts regarding code-switching and my insecurities towards speaking in my Trinidadian accent and dialect in university settings. I shared my sorrow existing in an academic space that lacked Black mentorship. I admitted to exchanging smiles with any Black person I met on campus, acknowledging that, though from diverse backgrounds, the commonalities I shared with other Black students were nestled within an *otherness* that was beyond our control. Panellists' familiarity with my encounters served as a motivator to instil a sense of safety and openness as they also shared their intimate thoughts about being Black in a dominating white space. I wanted the panellists to understand that they belong and are valued as students and in the future as faculty or staff if they choose to pursue such paths.

Dissemination can be an integral component when facilitating ethical discourse, as it allows participants' stories to be heard in various forums, thus strengthening marginalized voices. Freire (2002) emphasized the need for persons taking up leadership roles to alleviate oppression and work alongside oppressed persons when voicing the need for change. Assisting panellists to disseminate their views created avenues for our discussion to transcend the confines of the panel event. Brown and Danaher (2017) urged persons engaging in ethical facilitation to disseminate findings in manners that accentuate respect for and appreciation of participants. With a university professor's assistance, we created two short videos to highlight two significant issues arising from the discussion. The first video emphasized panellists' responses to the lack of Black professors and mentors at the university. The second focused on panellists' opinions regarding the lack of anti-racism or Black studies at their university. With panellists' approval, I capitalized on my position as a Black PhD student and the graduate student representative in the President's Bi Campus Committee for Equity, Diversity, and Inclusion (EDI) to enlighten the university's staff and administrators about their practices that intentionally or unintentionally marginalize students. In these forums, I showed the videos to predominantly white cohorts. Armed with a total of 15 points arising from the panel discussions and the cellphilm workshops, and using my experiences as examples, I identified the various university practices that hinder Black students from genuinely enjoying a safer university space. To name a few, I highlighted students' experiences with varying levels of racial discrimination, their lack of exposure to the province's and Canada's Black history, their views that their university focuses on diversity but disregards inclusion, and the lack of Black mentors within their university. In the hope of taking my discussion beyond merely highlighting issues of concern, I provided suggestions on ways the university can create safer spaces and address racial issues affecting its Black students. For instance, I cited George Mwangi and Fries-Britt's suggestions for effective strategies that universities can utilize to increase cross-cultural communication, create greater within-group peer interactions in the Black student population, and alleviate feelings of isolation and loneliness among racialized students. These strategies include recognizing the heterogeneity among the university's Black students, thus creating opportunities for Black students to connect with other Black students from countries that spread throughout the African Diaspora; establishing formal and informal events that encourage dialogue between both groups about student issues; hiring Black staff; and celebrating Black students' successes.

A Pathway to Positive Transformation

Over the years, Canada has experienced steady growth in international student enrolment (Houshmand, Spanierman, & Tafarodi, 2014) and Atlantic Canada has capitalized on its universities' drive towards greater recruitment of international students (Donovan, 2019) as a means of retaining a well-educated workforce (MSVU, 2019). Increasing numbers of Black international students are now pursuing education in provinces like New Brunswick. I possess first-hand experiences with the numerous challenges Black international students face. Black students must find solace in recognizing and emulating their forefathers' strength and resilience. Black people have demonstrated their strength and determination throughout history and proved that dehumanizing a race cannot cripple their desire and ability to lead. I implore local and international Black university students to follow our forefather's footsteps and heed the call for solidarity and advocacy. Embrace your privilege as emerging scholars and use your position in academic spaces to dismantle the erasure of Black stories and focus.

Although Black students in Canada are working towards self-empowerment, Canada's higher education institutions must also be intentional in creating inclusive environments for all students. Students' sense of connectedness with their school community can impact their success and overall well-being (Jones & Kim, 2020). Universities must adapt to students' varying geographics and demographics, and include staff and faculty to reflect these diversities. They must embrace the heterogeneous makeup of their student bodies and dismantle homogeneous academia to create a more inclusive, diverse institutional ethos. Jones and Kim (2020) posited that the United States and Canadian universities should be more intentional in providing for international students by facilitating multicultural mentoring programmes. These student activities foster solid relationships and cultural orientation, and train faculty in cultural humility. Anti-racism must form part of universities' systemic processes and classroom pedagogies. Canada's educators must engage students in discussions about racism. When educators guide students to explore racism and discrimination, they facilitate multicultural, anti-racist, and equitable learning environments. Only when these anti-racist initiatives become integral to Canada's universities and societies can Black students experience transformation towards more diverse, inclusive safe spaces.

Conclusion

This chapter provided an autoethnographic account of my journey to self-identity. I never realized I was Black until I entered a white space. Brand

(2001) wrote of a metaphorical *door of no return*. To her, it represented both a place in the imagination and a point in history – the Middle Passage that brought slaves to Trinidad. For me, this door of no return signifies my journey to the Canadian landscape. An identity that became part of me from the moment I entered the airplane destined for Canada. I can never again return to my previous identity as merely a woman who has overcome many challenges in life. I am now a *Black* woman who has and continues to overcome life challenges.

It is imperative that Black women and other minorities engage in academic activities that appropriately represent them and provide counternarratives to the hegemonic representations of whiteness as the norm (Hernandez et al., 2015). Through African Canadian feminist autoethnography, I contribute to the growing number of powerful Black women seeking to dismantle anti-Black racism and amplify Black women's voices in academia. Like me, junior scholars have the power to utilize anti-oppressive praxis through their writing to disrupt, challenge, and resist injustices masked with normality. As Lorenz (2018) emphasized, "In gifting our experiences to the world through our words, we can disseminate ideas and discourses that challenge the hierarchical norms of Canadian society. In so doing, we are writing resistance" (p. 7). I call on my Black colleagues to remain visible, recognize your privilege as scholars, and continue to engage in ethical discourse as a point of resistance.

Notes

1 In this chapter, I use the term *Black* to signify persons of African origin who formed part of the African Diaspora. Synonymous with Wane, Deliovsky, and Lawson's (2002) approach, I use the terms *African Canadian* and *Black* interchangeably to signify a person of African descent who resides in Canada.
2 Trinidad and Tobago's local music that forms a significant aspect of the country's carnival celebrations.

References

Backhouse, C. (1999). *Colour-coded: A legal history of racism in Canada, 1900–1950*. University of Toronto Press.
Baldwin, A., Cameron, L., & Kobayashi, A. (Eds.). (2012). *Rethinking the Great White North: Race, nature, and the historical geographies of Whiteness in Canada*. UBC Press.
Brand, D. (2001). *A map to the door of no return*. Doubleday Canada.
Brown, A., & Danaher, P. A. (2017). CHE principles: Facilitating authentic and dialogical semi-structured interviews in educational research. *International Journal of Research and Method in Education*, 42(1), 76–90. https://doi.org/10.1080/1743727X.2017.1379987
Cudjoe, S. R. (2017, July 02). State capture: Syrian/Lebanese style. *Trinidad and Tobago News Blog*. Retrieved from http://www.trinidadandtobagonews.com/blog/?p=10146

Donovan, M. (2019, April 15). Universities spend big on recruiters in scramble for foreign students. *CBC News*. Retrieved from https://www.cbc.ca/news/canada/nova-scotia/atlantic-canada-universities-recuiters-contracts-freedom-of-information-1.5095883

Freire, P. (2002). *Pedagogy of the oppressed* (50th anniversary ed.). The Continuum International Publishing Group.

Graham, A., Powell, M. A., & Truscott, J. (2016). Facilitating student well-being: Relationships do matter. *Educational Research, 58*(4), 366–383. https://doi.org/10.1080/00131881.2016.1228841

Gulliver, T. (2018). Canada the redeemer and denials of racism. *Critical Discourse Studies, 15*(1), 68–86. https://doi.org/10.1080/17405904.2017.1360192

Hébert, P. (2016). "70: Remembering a revolution" in Trinidad and Tobago. *Black Perspectives*. Retrieved from https://www.aaihs.org/70-remembering-a-revolution-in-trinidad-and-tobago/

Henry, A. (2015). 'We especially welcome applications from members of visible minority groups': Reflections on race, gender and life at three universities. *Race, Ethnicity and Education, 18*(5), 589–610. https://doi.org/10.1080/13613324.2015.1023787

Henry, F., & Tator, C. (2012). Interviews with racialized faculty members in Canadian universities. *Canadian Ethnic Studies, 44*(2), 75–99. https://doi.org/10.1353/ces.2012.0003

Hernandez, K. C., Ngunjiri, F. W., & Chang, H. (2015). Exploiting the margins in higher education: A collaborative autoethnography of three foreign born female faculty of color. *International Journal of Qualitative Studies in Education, 28*(5), 533–551. https://doi.org/10.1080/09518398.2014.933910

Hill, D. C., Callier, D. M., & Waters, H. L. (2019). Notes on terrible educations: Auto/ethnography as intervention to how we see Black. *Qualitative Inquiry, 25*(6), 539–543. https://doi.org/10.1177/1077800418806609

hooks, b. (1981). *Ain't I a woman: Black women and feminism*. South End Press.

hooks, b. (1994). *Teaching to transgress: Education as the practice of freedom*. Routledge.

Houshmand, S., Spanierman, L. B., & Tafarodi, R. W. (2014). Excluded and avoided: Racial microaggressions targeting Asian international students in Canada. *Cultural Diversity and Ethnic Minority Psychology, 20*(3), 377–388. Retrieved from https://psycnet.apa.org/doi/10.1037/a0035404

IS T&T, (2017, July 2). *Unacceptable to response Parts Unknown Trinidad* [Video]. YouTube. https://www.youtube.com/watch?v=cM-Az9EOqGY

Jones, A. H., & Kim, Y. K. (2020). The role of academic self-confidence on thriving among international college students in U.S. and Canada. *Journal of Underrepresented and Minority Progress, 4*(2), 165–191. https://doi.org/10.32674/jump.v4i2.2196

Kelley, R. D. G. (2018). Black study, Black struggle. *Ufahamu: A Journal of African Studies, 40*(2), 153–168. https://doi.org/10.5070/F7402040947

King, L. J. (2020). Black history is not American history: Toward a framework of Black historical consciousness. *Social Education 84*(6), 335–341.

Lorde, A. (2019). *Sister outsider: Essays and speeches*. Penguin Classics.

Lorenz, D. E. (2018). Pedagogies of resistance: Living resistance by writing. *Canadian Journal of New Scholars in Education*, 6–14. Retrieved from https://cjc-rcc.ucalgary.ca/index.php/cjnse/article/view/52970

MacEntee, K., Burkholder, C., & Schwab-Cartas, J. (2016). What's a cellphilm? An introduction. In K. MacEntee, C. Burkholder, & J. Schwab-Cartas (Eds.), *What's a cellphilm? Integrating mobile phone technology into participatory visual research activism* (pp. 1–15). Sense Publishers.

Marx, S., Pennington, J. L., & Chang, H. (2017). Critical autoethnography in pursuit of educational equity: Introduction to the IJME special issue. *International Journal of Multicultural Education, 19*(1), 1–6. http://doi.org/10.18251/ijme .v19i1.1393

Mathinenson, G. (2002). Reconceptualizing our classroom practice: Notes from an anti-racist educator. In N. N. Wane, K. Deliovsky, & E. Lawson (Eds.), *Back to the drawing board: African-Canadian feminism* (pp. 129–157). Sumach Press.

McCarthy, M. L. (2006). *Releasing my critical chatter: An autobiographical narrative from a Black diaspora* [Doctoral dissertation, University of New Brunswick]. Library and Archives Canada. https://central.bac-lac.gc.ca/.item?id=MR49705 &op=pdf&app=Library&oclc_number=697933057

McCarthy, M. L. (2014). Mixed-race identity Black and Maliseet. *Acadiensis, 43*(1), 117–124. Retrieved from https://id.erudit.org/iderudit/acad43_1for02

Mekonen, S. A. (2021). I am Black now: A phenomenologically grounded autoethnography of becoming Black in Berlin. In M. Kohl (Ed.), *Under construction: Performing critical identity* (pp. 9–28). MDPI.

Mensah, J. (2010). *Black Canadians: History, experience, social conditions.* Fernwood Publishing.

Mogadime, D. (2002). Black women in graduate studies: Transforming the socialization experience. In N. N. Wane, K. Deliovsky, & E. Lawson (Eds.), *Back to the drawing board: African-Canadian feminism* (pp. 129–157). Sumach Press.

Mohamed, T., & Beagan, B. L. (2019). Strange faces' in the academy: Experiences of racialized and indigenous faculty in Canadian universities. *Race, Ethnicity and Education, 22*(3), 338–354. https://doi.org/10.1080/13613324.2018 .1511532

Noreiga, A. F. (2020, February 6). Unearthing Black identities and feelings of isolation in Fredericton. *NB Media Co-op.* Retrieved from https://nbmediacoop.org/2020 /02/06/unearthing-black-identities-and-feelings-of-isolation-in-fredericton/

Noreiga, A. F. (in press). Facilitating Black identity and advocacy: Creating cellphilms for reflection on issues affecting Black university students. *Visual Studies.*

Noreiga, A. F., & Justin, S. (2021). A duo-ethnography of Black international university students in Canada. *Antistasis, 11*(1), 17–25. Retrieved from https:// journals.lib.unb.ca/index.php/antistasis/article/view/32309

Osei, K. (2019). Fashioning my garden of solace: A Black feminist autoethnography. *Fashion Theory, 23*(6), 733–746. https://doi.org/10.1080/1362704X.2019 .1657272

Rambo, C., & Ellis, C. (2020). Autoethnography. *The Blackwell Encyclopedia of Sociology,* 1–3. http://doi.org/10.1002/9781405165518.wbeosa082.pub2

Reynolds, G. (2016). *Viola Desmond's Canada: A history of Blacks and racial segregation in the promised land.* Fernwood Publishing.

Singleton, P. (2020). Remodelling Barbie, making justice: An autoethnography of craftivist encounters. *Feminism and Psychology,* 1–19. https://doi.org/10.1177 /0959353520941355

Spray, W. A. (1972). *The Blacks in New Brunswick.* St. Thomas University.

Sweet, J (Director). (2017, June 18). Trinidad (Season 9, Episode 7) [TV series episode]. In Anthony Bourdain: *Parts Unknown*. Zero Point Zero Production Inc.

The Roestone Collective. (2014). Safe space: Towards a reconceptualization. *Antipode*, 46(5), 1346–1365. https://doi.org/10.1111/anti.12089

Walker, J. W. G. (1985). *Racial discrimination in Canada: The Black experience*. The Canadian Historical Association.

Wane, N. N. (2002). Black-Canadian feminist thought: Drawing on the experiences of my sisters. In N. N. Wane, K. Deliovsky, & E. Lawson (Eds.), *Back to the drawing board: African-Canadian feminism* (pp. 129–157). Sumach Press.

Wane, N. N., Deliovsky, K., & Lawson, E. (2002). Introduction. In N. N. Wane, K. Deliovsky, & E. Lawson (Eds.), *Back to the drawing board: African-Canadian feminism* (pp. 129–157). Sumach Press.

8 Passing the Grade

Experiences of Black Males in Secondary Schools in Ontario, Canada

Daniel Lumsden

Introduction

The questioning, criticizing, and challenging of our education system is as critical today as it was during the legalization of racially segregated schools. As a former Black student attending a Toronto high school in the early '90s, and currently a Black educator in the city, I see and experience a tiered education system based on race. Black students do not have the same educational opportunities and experiences as their white student peers. Their interactions and relationships with their teachers are for the most part, incomparable. The subtle and sometimes unintentional acts of discrimination that Black students encounter daily can make their school experiences unpleasant, harmful, and paralyzing. The stories and experiences that we hear today from Black students resemble that of my own experiences and those of my friends going back three decades and more. As a Black educator I want to better understand these experiences and more importantly why Black students continue to feel like they do not belong in schools and do not feel valued or worthy to take a seat alongside their white student counterparts despite Ontario's "award-winning" Equity and Inclusive Education Strategy that launched in 2009. I wanted to know how Black male educators conceptualize what they experienced in secondary school and how they can reach out to Black students in their role as educators. With this in mind, this chapter will explore real-life experiences from three Black male educators as they reflect on Black student–teacher relationships and microaggressions that target Black male students in an education setting. These lived experiences offer to contextualize the issues Black male students and educators encounter and how these issues transcend over decades. Practical strategies will be provided to help uplift the experiences of Black males in our secondary schools.

My Position

My connection to this work as a Black male educator is real and validates my own personal and professional experiences and those that I have heard

DOI: 10.4324/9781003205296-10

along the way. I have learned that as Black males we shared the same experiences in high school regardless of where we attended high school – public or independent schools. I want all students, especially Black males to feel represented and have a sense of belonging within the school environment. I strive to help Black students believe in themselves and to keep their heads high at all times. They need to be told that regardless of what the world throws at us – they matter, we matter, us Black men matter.

While I have seen small changes that are starting to happen, I am not sure that the needle has been moved much. I also believe that we need more representation in educational leadership positions. We need to look at potential teacher bias and how that is reflected in the teaching of Black students and how we engage in developing relationships with Black students. While teacher education programmes may introduce issues such as bias, stereotypes, and racism, the school culture needs to prioritize how it will respond to these issues in their practice. One day I had someone tell me we need an all-Black university in Canada. It was a friend of mine that stated, "NO! We need current universities in our country to teach about Black history and introduce these courses in their programs. We need to look at the Eurocentric focus in our schools and curriculum and embed what Black Canadians and Indigenous Canadians have contributed to this land, and tell the real story." The truth is that this has remained hidden and denied over the years and must be exposed at all levels in education. We need courses to teach our students the contributions Black and Indigenous people have made to help shape this country, and to speak about colonization and how that is part of our history and can be seen today in systems and policies we are all trying to navigate in – some more easily than others. The opportunity for faculty and students to think critically and learn how to ask catalytic questions that will form the basis of great discourse in education. These conversations will hopefully reframe what they know about history and help to construct knowledge that is more inclusive and representative of Canadian history.

We often hear the excuse that this learning can only happen in our history classes. But I disagree. We can speak to this in any course. It just requires teachers to unlearn what they know to be true; to be innovative and find opportunities to embed these conversations in their courses. For example, in math and science we can speak about contributions Black people made to these subjects and advancements in the field. In business we can look at the economic class systems and how they came about, along with the power of big businesses and how they monopolize profits in poorer countries.

We have to disrupt education and the curriculum, because our Black students are not being represented, heard, or seen. I have always believed in the stance of changing the curriculum, so all students are being represented, and feel part of the learning environment. Many students have shared their disdain towards the book *To Kill a Mockingbird* and the use of the N-word leaving Black students feeling uncomfortable. As well, the lack of discussions in the classroom to elevate the moral complexities of the story that can still be seen in present day leave students questioning the value of this aspect of the curriculum. Again, if nothing is raised about this issue, our students will always feel ignored and remain marginalized. Having these conversations with peers inside and outside of school, several schools are no longer introducing this book in their classrooms. The importance of allyship in education is important, and sometimes having discourse with educators can make a difference. That does not mean the issues have been eliminated, but it is a step in the right direction.

A close friend of mine stated, "the train has left the station," but we remind ourselves that there is no such thing as a LAST STOP! The train must keep on moving and it starts with education. It is not up to me to educate others, but if we dismantle the Eurocentric values of our education system by speaking up, and teaching all students how to think critically, to see their education as a way to make positive social changes in our world and for all people living in our world, then we will move the needle. One way to accomplish this progress is through allyship from the dominant group and solidarity amongst our marginalized groups of people. While there is a small group of people in the caboose of the train that is reluctant to move up – to truly see the new tracks being laid out in front of it, the train continues to move forward. We must continue to move forward.

Canada's History with Racism

The reason, whether or not we wish to admit it, is that Canada has a long history of racism towards Indigenous and Black people. Canada had already enslaved many African people in the early seventeenth century (Whitfield, 2020). The Maritimes, which is located in the Eastern part of Canada, consists of three provinces: Nova Scotia, New Brunswick, and Prince Edward Island. According to Whitfield (2020), the enslavement of Black people is part of the history of the Canadian Maritimes. Black slaves in the Maritimes were referred to as either a *free* Black or a Black *slave* (Whitfield, 2007), and someone labelled as a free Black lived fearing that they could be re-enslaved or sold back to the West Indies at any time and for any reason that their white counterparts might find threatening, offensive, or disloyal. Black slaves from the United States who were seeking freedom were brought to Canada through the Underground Railway, a network of people who wanted to do away with slavery and help African American slaves escape to Northern States in the United States or Canada (Wigmore, 2011). This narrative of Canada being a haven (Hepburn, 1999) for Black slaves from the United States has been the main story told and retold to illustrate Canada's connection to Black slavery, while glazing over its own involvement in enslaving Black people and upholding a system that would never truly recognize Black people as free and equal members of its nation.

Education System

In the Canadian education system, students start as young as the age of 4 when they enter junior kindergarten and complete elementary school by grade 8 (age 13). High school or secondary school in the Canadian context starts at grade 9 and ends in grade 12 (age 18), where students usually move on to post-secondary education. The Ontario system consists of a public secular board that includes English and Catholic boards, and a public separate board that includes an English Catholic board, French Catholic board, and an English Protestant board. Both the public secular and public separate school boards receive funding from the provincial governments. The Ontario education system also has independent schools that could start as early as junior and senior kindergarten and move up to grade 12. These schools are fee-based with an annual tuition determined by the individual school that students must pay to attend. The independent schools receive no funding from the government but are mandated to follow the Ontario curriculum. Ontario's publicly funded schools make education accessible and remove cost as a barrier to accessing education.

The architecture of the education system is not being challenged; it is how the system is wired that I am attempting to expose. The end to racially segregated schools did not necessarily result in an end to the racism or oppressive acts towards Black students. Today, systemic racism and oppression within the educational context plays out in different ways via streaming and expulsions/suspensions.

Despite the Ontario Ministry of Education and Training's update to the 1993 Policy/Program Memorandum (PPM) No. 119 to include policies for anti-racism and ethnocultural equality, Black students continue to feel under-represented, discriminated, and not heard or seen as students or future contributors to society. Historically, Black students underperformed due to the disenfranchisement in urban school settings and the inequity structures in our schools (Lomotey & Lowery, 2014). The province of Ontario has the largest diverse ethnic makeup out of all the provinces in Canada (Tuters & Portelli, 2017). There has been great population growth with regard to people of colour and students of colour; however, this same growing population continually reports that the schools do not represent them or their experiences. Dei et al. (2003) mention that students whose first language is not English often do not experience the same academic achievements as students in the dominant culture. However, there are countries within the Caribbean where English is predominantly the first language of the people and yet Robyn Maynard (2017) states that "in Quebec, students with Caribbean backgrounds are three times more likely to be identified as students with handicaps, social maladjustments or learning difficulties and subsequently placed in separate classes for 'at risk' students" (p. 215). Maynard goes on to explain that this classification allows for school officials to have discretionary power of who gets labelled with this designation and how they are to be treated. The creation and adoption of such policies look a lot like racial profiling and streaming of Black students without any further evaluation or measurement to assess the potential for learning difficulties.

Maynard (2017) notes other examples of racial profiling and academic streaming calling out a significant over-representation of Black students in Halifax having individual programme plans (IPPs), and in a diverse city like Toronto where only 3% of Black students are designated as "gifted," but make up 13% of the student body. Compare this to their white student peers in Toronto who make up nearly one-third of the student population, and over half are designated as "gifted" (Maynard, 2017).

A report completed by Colour of Poverty – Colour of Change (2019), an organization network across the province of Ontario, mentioned of those students taking academic-level courses in 2015 with the Toronto District School Board (TDSB), meaning they have a pathway to go to university or college, 53% of Black students were represented compared to 81% of their white student counterparts. When we look at expulsion within the TDSB, Black students only make up 12% of the population but received 48% of the expulsions within the board (Colour of Poverty – Colour of Change, 2019). These are examples in Ontario of racially profiling Black students, streaming Black students onto a path that limits their academic options following secondary school, and imposing harsher disciplinary measures onto these students. These are the decisions made by the system that continue to oppress our Black students and are the narratives that need to be told.

Layered onto racial profiling and the streaming of Black students, these students often face racism, homophobia, and other forms of oppression and microaggressions (Tuters & Portelli, 2017). Codjoe (2001) stated the education experience of Black students is one where they experience harm and psychological violence. While Ontario's education system has dissolved racially segregated schools in the interest of the white Eurocentric dominant group, racial discrimination and inequality remain within the system. They are woven into policies, whether intentional or not, and are reflected in practice creating a detrimental imbalance, based on race, to an educational experience that should offer equal access to educational opportunities and a safe, inclusive space to learn.

Critical Race Theory

Critical race theory (CRT) is often used in education to distinguish the inequalities of oppressed groups. It is a theoretical framework that was evolved in the 1980s by legal scholars to help us realize how racial disparities live through in our society and how that gives rise to some of our laws and policies. Delgado and Stefancic (2012) mention CRT is "a collection of activists and scholars interested in studying and trans-forming the relationship among race, racism, and power" (p. 3). Delgado and Stefancic also state that critical race theory is based around four tenants: race is ordinary – not aberrational, material determinism, social construction, and a unique voice of colour. Recently Bonila-Silva (2015) redeveloped the tenants set out by Delgado and Stefancic and adapted the following: Racism is embedded in the structure of society; racism has a psychology; racism changes over different times; racism has a degree of rationality: overt, covert, and normative racialized behaviours; and racism has a contemporary foundation. Despite 20 years of research completed by Bonila-Silva and other critical race theorists, we are still faced today with the notion of oppression of minority groups in our society.

Acts of racism, racial inequality, and discrimination are seen in the streaming of racialized students as described earlier in this chapter, the under-representation of racialized students, and the microaggressions they endure on a daily basis that go unnoticed because the discriminatory beliefs towards minority groups have been normalized throughout the years.

Anti-racism initiatives in education challenges administrations, educators, and students to examine the role white supremacy plays in education and society as a whole, and in the privilege assigned to white people that puts non-white people at a disadvantage because of race alone. Teaching anti-racism in education can help students to recognize racism as a social, systemic construct that can feel subtle or non-existent to some, while for others it is crude, obvious, and true to life.

Social justice in education looks at both the actions and practices of inequality within the system and its structure within the classrooms. For example, the development of the curriculum is the responsibility of the school board, the governing system and structure for all education across the province, which determines the curriculum to be taught in the classroom. When Indigenous and Black people are represented in the curriculum, it is a publicly recognized day or month, like Indigenous Peoples' Day or Black History Month. The criticism to education in regard to these attempts of diversity and inclusion is that the content tends to be fixated on the acts of "past" oppression with hesitancy to accept and engage in healthy discourse about race, and racial oppression and inequalities that exist today. Racialized and non-racialized students are not learning about the positive contributions made by members of Black, Indigenous, and People of Colour (BIPOC) communities, therefore creating barriers for racialized students to engage with the curriculum in a way that is meaningful and represents their history, experiences, and values. Whether intentional or not, the absence of critical dialogue in education about race, racism, and oppression allows for the white dominant group to tell and retell history from their white, Eurocentric perspective. These stories have grossly misled people about the true identities of Blacks, Indigenous, and People of Colour, and continue to keep the status quo of the white dominant culture in power and the oppression of BIPOC communities. If we do not use education to facilitate these critical discussions and work to unlearn our history, then we are only contributing to the pain and suffering of Black, Indigenous, and People of

Colour causing more harm. As an educator, I do not see this profession as a mechanism used to oppress; I see it as a catalyst for positive change and personal freedom.

The Brazilian philosopher Paulo Freire was a critical educator and may be considered a founder of critical pedagogy (Giroux, 2010). Freire (1970) in his book *Pedagogy of the Oppressed* criticizes educators and the system for encouraging students to assume a passive role in their education. Freire describes the teacher-centred approach through what he coined the term "banking concept," meaning the system valued the teacher as the keeper of all knowledge and the students were empty vessels. The teacher deposits knowledge onto these "empty"-minded students, which results in students learning (Freire, 1970). The content to be learned is constructed for the students based on the teacher's idea of what is relevant and hinders any opportunity for intellectual growth. Rugat and Osman (2013) add to Freire's banking concept by stating that this approach results in students being fed information from their instructor with the expectation that students simply memorize the information. This perspective of traditional instruction places the teacher as the expert, giving the teacher full power of the content being taught, while the students are receivers of this knowledge. Freire challenged the education system and educators to revolutionize education through the practice of critical pedagogy, promoting the co-learning and co-creation of knowledge with teachers and students together through relevant problem-posing education models. The fundamental underpinnings in Freire's critical pedagogy are for the "development of critical consciousness, which enables learners to recognize connections between their individual problems and experiences and the social contexts in which they are embedded" (Nylund & Tilsen, 2006, p. 22).

Critical Pedagogy

Critical pedagogy is inspired by critical theory and challenges us to examine how education can best be offered to all students. Critical pedagogy looks at social justice, agency, and privilege, and encourages opportunities for students to question domination, and the beliefs and practices that perpetuate the domination of one group over other groups. Critical pedagogy should be a concern for all educators. Murrell (1997, p. 23) asks, "Can schooling for African-American children ever be more than institutional indoctrination into a social system and American culture that reproduces, reinforces and fortifies the devaluation of African-American people?" For people who are marginalized in society, Freire believes the initial step regarding their transformation is the ability to see themselves in their current situation as it relates to the institutional and social constructs that have been set in place, and to have the tools to better redefine those constructs and how they interact within them.

Methods

I set out to explore and attempt to learn more about how Black male educators conceptualize what they were exposed to in secondary school and how they can reach out to Black students. Personally and professionally I thought this work would connect me with other teachers who had similar questions, experiences of hardships and suffering, and maybe even together, had some ideas for solutions. The interviews conducted with three Black male educators and shared within this chapter aim to raise awareness of racial issues in education, create urgency to necessitate everyone's contribution to addressing these issues, and attempt to validate the Black student and educator experience and the systematic suffering while attending their respective institutions.

Participants

The next section of this chapter will dive into experiences from three Black Ontario educators who reflected on their own high school careers and how they use their experiences to reach out to Black students in their schools (Table 8.1). A purposeful sample (Cresswell, 2012) was used to have a better understanding of who could participate. The recruitment of my participants was deliberate in nature. The following criteria were selected: (1) participants had to be certified educators teaching in K–12 schools, and (2) they had to identify as Black males. All interviews with participants took place in the year 2020 in a face-to-face format that lasted for one hour for each participant. Further interviews were also conducted after more questions arrived from the findings, and those interviews ranged from 30 minutes to 1 hour. It is important to note that interviews were conducted offsite, and all interviews were transcribed from audio recordings.

Relationships

There is this uncertain truth that Black male students generally do not do as well as their white counterparts in an education setting. These thoughts have a way of being internalized by Black male students, impacting their performance in school and their relationships with their teachers. Dei (2008) would attest that parents have to be involved in the motivation of students'

Table 8.1 Teacher Participants

Secondary Educator	Years of Service	Ethnicity
Andrew	25	Black
Michael	17	Black
David	19	Black

success, along with the students' connection with educators and other stake-holders in the school environment in order to gain and enhance the success of Black students. Mental health plays an important role in some of our students, and one area mentioned by Legette et al. (2020) is social and emotional learning, and their importance to relationship skills plays a vital part in the success of Black students. Healthy relationships are vital to a student's overall well-being. When speaking with fellow Black male educators about their relationships with Black teachers they may have had throughout their schooling, one thing seemed quite evident: there are few Black educators. Only one (Andrew) out of the three participants interviewed was taught by a Black educator – a male educator in secondary school. The general experience of Black students back then was that many did not see Black educators until they went onto post-secondary schooling. Black educator representation was more common in post-secondary than in secondary school, yet still disproportionate to their white colleagues. It is important that Black students have teachers that look like them, see them, and can speak for them. One teacher described the importance of affinity that is present between Black educators and Black students, and that it can boost a student's sense of belonging when they see themselves reflected in faculty.

Another educator, David, who identifies as Black and has been teaching at the secondary school level in Ontario for 19 years, spoke about his role in enhancing the experience of Black students and their relationships with each other and with other Black educators at the school. He and a fellow teacher brought forward the idea of a space for Black students, by Black students, bringing together Black students and Black teachers to connect and share experiences in and outside of school. This was their space after school. Once a week, Black students that belonged to this group met with several Black teachers, and discussed what problems they were facing or spoke about issues in society all together. What was key to this group was that these students needed accessibility. They needed a place where they could vent their frustrations and have the support of everyone in the room. One of the challenges of creating this initiative was student buy-in. David spoke about how difficult it was at first to get students to attend meetings because of the extracurricular schedules. David and another colleague had to choose a date where they made it mandatory for Black students to attend the session. When they shared with the Black students the purpose of the affinity group, that was enough for students to see the benefits of his group. When the group was formed, white teachers wanted to know why a meeting was being held for Black students after school. White colleagues asked if the students were being disciplined and what did they do? They even had a teacher interrupt their meeting, pretending they were looking for something in their classroom, because they wanted to overhear the conversations. Another challenge was having colleagues asking to join their group that did not identify as Black. The Black students did not feel comfortable sharing their thoughts and experiences with these teachers, for fear of receiving a bad grade or being treated differently in the classroom. These examples really amplify evidence presented earlier about racial profiling and stereotyping that Black students face daily. While these may seem like insignificant acts, they are a constant reminder of the struggle that Black students face even when they are just trying to belong. The opportunity for these students to come together, and the importance of having this affinity group for students from grades 9 to 10 was explained by David:

> It is obvious Black students needed a place where they could vent and be heard. I believe that having Black educators in the school – they feel safe around us, and more importantly they trust us. The students often speak about a multitude of things from the microaggressions they face in school, to their home environment, and issues going on in the world. More importantly, they tell us they look up to us, and are thankful that we are here. This often transcends into the classroom, knowing that they are part of this environment and feel that their voice is heard.

These Black educators are co-creating a space for Black students to feel free to speak their minds and learn how to respond when faced with microaggression statements made towards them. They are teaching students how to be respectful, but challenge a person whom they feel made a microaggression towards them.

Facilitating these groups takes careful consideration. It is an outlet for Black students to share their experiences from the most painful to the most joyous. Ensuring that these groups are not focused on deficit-based thinking is a consideration that facilitators like David need to keep in mind. The term *deficit thinking* only focuses on the hardships that students may have encountered up until now (Martin et al., 2018). While this group does focus on the hardships, as it is important to discuss these issues, this Black affinity group also looks at the potential in these students. David acknowledges the group focuses on the successes of the students, and has invited Black guest speakers from various industries to speak to students about what skills they are looking for in hiring candidates. The group also provides materials for post-secondary education and what courses will be needed along with post-secondary schools that may interest them. Finally, the group will speak to coping mechanisms when dealing with hardships and how to move on from them in a positive way.

While speaking with Black educators it was evident that Black students know if you are in their corner or not. Once they know that you are in their corner, they will generally start to open up about themselves. Speaking with the participants, this is mainly achieved outside the classroom. Black students have told the participants it is as easy as giving them a fist bump, a simple gesture to acknowledge them in the hallways – even if an educator may not know them. Participants also noted that communicating to Black students that you are around and available to answer questions about classwork, or anything else they may have questions about. It provides a sense of appreciation and understanding of the connection between Black male teachers and Black students. One teacher (Michael) shared that it is important to strengthen these relationships with these students because we want them to be prepared for their next chapter in their life. He was very adamant about the success of Black students. He mentioned that we need a school position called BIPOC success support. He further explained why we needed a position of this sort for Black students, and especially Black males:

> Black students are for the most part not part of the conversations their white counterparts (peers) are having at the dinner table when it comes to post-secondary schooling, or connections to internships, or summer jobs. It is imperative that Black students are given the tools and skills needed to attend University or College, and what course/steps they need to take to be competitive. That starts with where to volunteer, where to apply for an internship, what skills are workplaces looking for in people working at their organization. What technology skills do these students need? If they are given the same blueprint as their white peers, our [Black] students will be that much more prepared and competitive.

It could be argued that the role of a guidance counsellor can help to provide that roadmap or boost student preparedness for post-secondary life. The reality here is the same issues apply. Black students are stereotyped to be less academically inclined than their white student peers. Academic courses offered in Ontario schools are considered the most challenging option in the secondary school curriculum ahead of applied and essential courses. A study conducted by the TDSB in 2015 showed that 39% of Black students compared to 16% of their white counterparts were likely to take applied-level courses (James & Turner, 2017). When we look at post-secondary acceptances, 25% of Black students confirmed acceptances, while students that identify as other racialized and white, comprised 60% and 47%, respectively (James & Turner, 2017). At the other end of the spectrum, 43% of Black students did not apply to university as compared to 17% and 26% of students who identified as other racialized and white, respectively (James and Turner, 2017).

One teacher shared experiences of Black students and the advice they received from their guidance counsellors. Black students have been advised to take non-university courses, or for Black students who expressed interest in applying to universities, they were steered towards applying for colleges. Some Black students have been advised to look into labour or construction jobs even after expressing a specific field of study at the university or college level.

Again we still have the same issues around Black representation among guidance counsellors. When we think of the ideal relationship between students and their guidance counsellors we often think about a relationship of trust, support, student-centred, and motivational. Are these the relationship characteristics that are present between Black students and their predominantly white guidance counsellors? If we see evidence in streaming that is race based, then there is systemic racism in our guidance system. In 2015, the TDSB reported that 9% of Black students were in essential courses, whereas that figure is three times larger than their white or other racialized peers (James & Turner, 2017). They further report that Black students in the TDSB compose 39% of students taking applied-level courses, compared to 18% and 16% by other racialized peers and white peers, respectively. Finally, academic courses report that 53% of Black students take academic courses, whereas other racialized and white peers composed 80% and 81%, respectively (James & Turner, 2017). The first step would be to conduct an audit of existing policies and practices of the guidance department through an anti-racism lens and commit to reform those policies and practices to ensure that we are addressing the disproportionate number of racialized students who are advised to take applied-level courses or lower. Professional learning grounded in the foundational underpinnings of anti-racism, anti-oppression, and anti-Black racism should be offered to staff as well as a reframing of their roles as guidance counsellors and their relationship in supporting racialized students.

Microaggressions

Microaggressions are a form of racial bias as insults directed towards minorities in an indirect way (Lilienfeld, 2017). When my three participants were asked to share their experiences on microaggressions, there was no shortage of examples that were provided:

- "Called the N-word."
- "That kid is a Jamaican and they are trouble."
- "Wow, you are so articulate in your explanations."
- "I do not see colour."
- "Racism does not exist here in Canada."

One of the teachers described a situation at a business function where he had taken several pieces of watermelon, when his superiors made a degrading comment about Black men and watermelon. He goes on to state, "This is several years ago, and we are still going through this."

Microaggressions can be explicit and can also be less obvious and hard to recognize. People sometimes attempt to disguise these hurtful comments as jokes or compliments, but the intention is to make the recipient feel inferior. Students experiencing microaggressions at school can have an increased level of stress and depression, and their academic performance can be negatively impacted (Ackerman-Barger et al., 2021). There is research that suggests that teachers are more likely to think their classes are too challenging for Black students and students of colour (Cherng, 2017). This perception is concerning and can be problematic to students when they feel that their abilities are being underestimated by their teacher, because they can internalize these lower expectations resulting in lower achievements (Cherng, 2017). These students are also likely to show signs of post-traumatic stress and are reported to likely engage in risky behaviours, such as drug and alcohol use, being involved in fights, and engaging in sexual activity, as a coping mechanism (Flores et al., 2010).

Strategies for Dismantling Systemic Racism

Following are three strategies that came out of the interviews, and address critical pedagogies moving forward with regards to relationships and microaggressions. The three strategies described are how to respond, inclusive and diversity training, and hiring practices.

How to Respond

From a critical pedagogy perspective we have to start deconstructing the policies and curriculum that help support racism. Reform in curriculum is past due. Our curriculum needs to embed knowledge and experiences across all subjects that will help dismantle discriminatory attitudes and beliefs. Education needs to embrace uncomfortable discourse. Students and faculty need to be able to identify aspects of the system that are supporting racism and oppression along with acts of microaggression. We need to all learn how to assert ourselves and call out these microaggressions and not avoid raising these issues with white people. These conversations may become uncomfortable, but these conversations are needed. Robin DiAngelo (2018) in her book *White Fragility* outlines how to give feedback to those who may be uncomfortable receiving it. She mentions using the proper tone is crucial to relaying your message, because it would be dismissed if the proper tone is not being used. DiAngelo also mentions feedback must be given immediately, because if we do not act on it right away, it will be discounted, and the behaviour and beliefs will perpetuate.

Professional Learning

Professional learning is important to supporting Ontario's Equity and Inclusive Education Strategy. We need to have training that focuses on diversity, inclusivity, and anti-racism. We have seen milestones regarding diversity, such as women in leadership roles, and multicultural representation in the workforce, but inclusion is still lagging. Dobbin et al. (2016) would agree that inclusion may be lacking, because when it comes to workplace questions, white people are taught how to take the tests and they soon forget about the biases a day or two after taking the company test. We need to embed training at the time of pre-service (teachers in training) and throughout their career to ensure that all teachers are well equipped to teach students from diverse backgrounds (James & Turner, 2017). Professional learning for teachers at all levels and even early childhood educators (pre-school) should be provided with education and training in anti-colonial and critical race theory with a special focus on anti-Black racism (James & Turner, 2017).

The challenging part of all of this from what I have seen is that these trainings are partially about increasing awareness and knowledge, and primarily about exploring our own values and implicit biases that support white supremacy. There has to be a growth mindset to unlearning what you think you know about the world around you and about your unconscious feelings and beliefs that support racism despite your best efforts to being an anti-racist.

Hiring Practices

Our schools need to better reflect the students attending these schools and the families that are part of the larger community. There is a gap in teacher diversity here in Ontario. According to Turner (2015), the Teacher Diversity Gap shows that in Ontario, the racialized population is 26%, while the percentage of teachers who are racialized is only 13%, thus having a large teacher diversity gap (.50). Turner sums up the findings by saying, "In terms of racial demographics, teachers in Ontario and Toronto Census Metropolitan Area (CMA) are far less diverse than the student population they teach" (p. 12). Turner further adds that with Canada's growing racialized population there is a case for the government to present to boards of education and independent schools, to prioritize the hiring of more racialized educators, and to create a school community that values inclusion and focuses on promoting inclusive practices that will benefit a diverse school body of students.

Black educator representation allows Black students to see themselves in the school, validating their place. The experiences Black educators can create for Black students in terms of affinity groups and brave spaces to talk is an important strategy to boost a sense of belonging and acceptance, and a strategy that cannot be easily duplicated without Black educators onboard.

Conclusion

It is clear that education can serve as a catalyst for change. Education can teach students to identify what needs to change in order for there to be equality for all, and how they can be agents of that change in the world. While government and educational institutions are making attempts to address issues around social justice within the system and in the schools, there are gaps in the practice of those same changes designed to act in response to issues of social justice in our education. There is an opportunity to look at the Black male teacher perspective on the role education plays in dismantling systemic racism and racial inequalities that only serve the best interest of the dominant white-European group. This will allow for the voices of Black educators to share what they think the barriers are to ending racism and opportunities to facilitate the end of racism through education and learning our way out of centuries of injustice.

References

Ackerman-Barger, K., Jacobs, N. N., Orozco, R., & London, M. (2021). Addressing microaggressions in academic health: A workshop for inclusive excellence. *MedEdPORTAL*, *17*(1), 11103–11103. https://doi.org/10.15766/mep_2374 -8265.11103

Bonilla-Silva, E. (2015). More than prejudice: Restatement, reflections, and new directions in critical race theory. *Sociology of Race and Ethnicity*, *1*(1), 73–87. https://doi-org.qe2a-proxy.mun.ca/10.1177/2332649214557042

Cherng, H.-Y. (2017). If they think I can: Teacher bias and youth of color expectations and achievement. *Social Science Research*, *66*, 170–186. https://doi .org/10.1016/j.ssresearch.2017.04.001

Codjoe, H. M. (2001). Fighting a 'Public enemy' of Black academic achievement-The persistence of racism and the schooling experiences of Black students in Canada. *Race, Ethnicity and Education*, *4*(4), 343–375. https://doi-org.qe2a-proxy.mun .ca/10.1080/13613320120096652

Colour of Poverty – Colour of Change. (2019). *Racialized poverty in education & learning: How are racialized people disadvantaged in education and learning?* [Fact Sheet]. Retrieved from https://colourofpoverty.ca/wp-content/uploads/2019 /03/cop-coc-fact-sheet-3-racialized-poverty-in-education-learning-3.pdf

Creswell, J. W. (2012). *Educational research: Planning, conducting, and evaluating quantitative and qualitative research* (4th ed.). Pearson Education.

Dei, G., James, I., Karumanchery, L., James-Wilson, S., & Zine, J. (2003). *Removing the margins: The challenges and possibilities of inclusive schooling*. Canadian Scholars' Press.

Delgado, R., & Stefancic, J. (2012). *Critical race theory: An introduction* (2nd ed.). New York University Press.

DiAngelo, R. (2018). *White fragility: Why it's so hard for white people to talk about racism*. Beacon Press.

Dobbin, F., & Kalev, A. (2016, July 08). Why diversity programs fail and what works better. *Harvard Business Review*. https://hbr.org/2016/07/ why-diversity-programs-fail

Flores, E., Tschann, J. M., Dimas, J. M., Pasch, L. A., & de Groat, C. L. (2010). Perceived racial/ethnic discrimination, posttraumatic stress symptoms, and health risk behaviors among Mexican American adolescents. *Journal of Counseling Psychology*, *57*(3), 264–273. https://doi.org/10.1037/a0020026

Freire, P. (1970). *Pedagogy of the oppressed*. Seabury Press.

Giroux, H. A. (2010). Rethinking education as the practice of freedom: Paulo Freire and the promise of critical pedagogy. *Policy Futures in Education*, *8*(6), 715–721.

Hepburn, S. A. R. (1999). Following the North Star: Canada as a haven for nineteenth-century American Blacks. *Michigan Historical Review, 25*(2), 91–126. https://doi.org/10.2307/20173830

James, C. E., & Turner, T. (2017). *Towards race equity in education: The schooling of Black students in the greater Toronto area.* York University.

Legette, K. B., Rogers, L. O., & Warren, C. A. (2020). Humanizing student–teacher relationships for Black children: Implications for teachers' social–emotional training. *Urban Education.* https://doi.org/10.1177/0042085920933319

Lilienfeld, S. O. (2017). Microaggressions: Strong claims, inadequate evidence. *Perspectives on Psychological Science, 12*(1), 138–169. https://doi.org/10.1177/1745691616659391

Lomotey, K., & Lowery, K. (2014). Black students, urban schools, and Black principals: Leadership practices that reduce disenfranchisement. In H. R. Milner & K. Lomotey (Eds.), *Handbook of urban education* (2nd ed., pp. 325–349). Routledge. Retrieved from https://doi-org.qe2a-proxy.mun.ca/10.4324/9780429331435

Martin, G. L., Smith, M. J., & Williams, B. M. (2018). Reframing deficit thinking on social class. *New Directions for Student Services, 162*(162), 87–93. https://doi-org.qe2a-proxy.mun.ca/10.1002/ss.20264

Maynard, R. (2017). *Policing Black lives: State violence in Canada from slavery to the present.* Fernwood.

Murrell, P. (1997). Chapter three: Digging again the family wells: A Freirian literacy framework as emancipatory pedagogy for African-American children. *Counterpoints, 60,* 19–58.

Nylund, D., & Tilsen, J. (2006). Pedagogy and praxis: Postmodern spirit in the classroom. *Journal of Systemic Therapies, 25*(4), 21–31. http://doi.org.qe2a-proxy.mun.ca/10.1521/jsyt.2006.25.4.21

Rugut, E. J., & Osman, A. A. (2013). Reflection on Paulo Freire and classroom relevance. *American International Journal of Social Science, 2*(2), 23–28.

Sefa Dei, G. J. (2008). Schooling as community: Race, schooling, and the education of African youth. *Journal of Black Studies, 38*(3), 346–366. https://doi.org/10.1177/0021934707306570

Turner, T. (2015). *Voices of Ontario Black educators: An experiential report.* Ontario Alliance of Black School Educators (ONABSE). Turner Consulting Group. Retrieved from http://onabse.org/ONABSE_VOICES_OF_BLACK_EDUCATORS_Final_Report.pdf

Tuters, S., & Portelli, J. (2017). Ontario school principals and diversity: Are they prepared to lead for equity? *The International Journal of Educational Management, 31*(5), 598–611. https://doi.org.qe2a-proxy.mun.ca/10.1108/IJEM-10-2016-0228

Whitfield, H. A. (2007). Black loyalists and Black slaves in Maritime Canada. *History Compass, 5*(6), 1980–1997. https://doi.org/10.1111/j.1478-0542.2007.00479

Whitfield, H. A. (2020). White archives, Black fragments: Problems and possibilities in telling the lives of enslaved Black people in the Maritimes. *The Canadian Historical Review, 101*(3), 323–345. https://doi.org/10.3138/chr-2019-0050

Wigmore, G. (2011). Before the railroad: From slavery to freedom in the Canadian-American borderland. *Journal of American History, 98*(2), 437–454.

Part 3

Forgetting as Pedagogy

When we experience pain and trauma, it often evokes strong emotions and feelings. In such circumstances, forgetting can be used as a survival and coping mechanism to avoid being retraumatized. We forget so that we can survive. We forget so that we do not have to remember. We cannot minimize this. Forgetting is at times necessary for survival. We throw around statements such as "Time heals all wounds." Does it? Time is only one factor amongst many others such as access to a supportive community, caring relationships, and peaceful existence. Those who live in contexts where civil strife and repression are regular occurrences may not be able to process the ongoing pain they are experiencing. Similarly, forgetting is difficult when you are constantly being triggered by events such as the regular discovery of gravesites of Indigenous children in Canada or the anti-Black racism that leads to the deaths of Black men, women, and children in the United States.

We also know that we never truly ever completely forget. In some of my graduate research, I (Steve Sider) explored the science of language learning and language loss. I was intrigued with my own experience of speaking Hindi as my first language but forgetting much of it when my family moved to Canada. As I pursued my research, I discovered many others who had similar experiences. For example, I interviewed a person who had learned Spanish as a child, thought he had forgotten it but spoke it fluently while in a comatose state after an accident as an adult. Similarly, when I was the primary caregiver for my father-in-law when he was in the grips of advanced dementia, I was amazed at his memory for childhood events even though he did not know his own name. In my own experience, the Hindi language flowed back to me when I returned to India. I had not forgotten the language, but I had a difficulty in retrieving it. In this sense, we choose to remember so that we do not forget.

In somewhat similar ways, our experiences of pain and trauma are never completely forgotten. They remain even when we try to forget or work to suppress the painful memories. They may be manifested through dreams or nightmares. We may suddenly experience a flashback when a triggering event occurs. They can influence our relationships with our partners or children. We may define ourselves through the pain and trauma that we have

DOI: 10.4324/9781003205296-11

experienced, even if we are not aware that this is what we are doing. In my own experience of leaving home in one country and moving to another, and moving through half a dozen schools in as many years, I now look back and see how I became a chameleon. I masked the pain by becoming invisible, not drawing attention to myself, and withdrawing from anything that might cause me further pain.

So how can forgetting serve as a form of pedagogy? As teachers, we want to help our students build their learning. We want them to recall knowledge and skills, not forget these things. In this book, we posit that forgetting and remembering are both aspects of learning. Pain and trauma sometimes need to be forgotten because that is actually healthy. If we did not forget, we would not be able to continue the day-to-day activities of life. However, we never fully forget. The remembering process can also be a healing balm. It is through remembering that we process the pain and grief. If we did not have pain, we would not understand what it means to live without it. It is through remembering that we commit to a new way forward. It is through remembering that we engage with others who have experienced similar pain. It is through remembering that we help our students process their own painful experiences. Dwayne Donald (2013), an Indigenous author, states, "For teaching and learning to be meaningful, we need to see ourselves in ecological relation to that which we want to know. Relations always come first" (p. 19). Relationships are at the heart of teaching.

As teachers, we are part of a relational act. As such, the pedagogy we engage in must involve trust. Trust is built through vulnerability. The forgetting and remembering of painful experiences is what can help build trust between teachers and students. It pushes us into this ecological space that can remove barriers and see each other as humans. Donald (2013) continues by stating:

> Ethical relationality – an ecological understanding of human relationality that does not deny difference, but rather seeks to more deeply understand how our different histories and experiences position us in relation to each other. This form of relationality is ethical because it does not overlook or invisibilise the particular historical, cultural, and social contexts from which a standpoint arises. It puts these considerations at the forefront of engagements across frontiers of difference. (p. 19)

Forgetting and remembering are pedagogy because we all have experienced pain. We use this pain as a form of relationality that binds us together across differences. We can use painful events as lessons in classes, as opportunities to engage students who may be experiencing similar pain; in our writing and storytelling that centres our lived experiences; and in engaging in critical pedagogy which challenges the hegemonic systems that perpetuate pain and suffering. It is important to remember that people might not be ready to share their pain and that is OK too. We are all in a process of learning and understanding; likewise, forgetting as a form of pedagogy is a dynamic process that calls us into an ethical relationality that can serve as a foundational aspect of teaching and learning.

Reference

Donald, D. (2013). On making love to death: Plains Cree and Blackfoot wisdom. In M. Smith (Ed.), *Transforming the academy: Essays on indigenous education, knowledges and relations.* Canadian Federation for the Humanities and Social Sciences. (pp. 14–19).

9 Sacred Tears

Indigenous Women's Healing Journey of Mobilization for Educational Systemic Change

Sharla Mskokii Peltier and Charis Auger

Indigenous leaders, parents, students, and educators have lived experience of marginalization within formal educational institutions, which they believe have failed dismally to provide an environment and educational philosophy conducive to Indigenous student success (Battiste, 1998; Dion, 2009; Henderson, 2012). The residential school system is an artefact of racism and colonialism within the educational system, reflecting the privilege of Euro-Canadian knowledge and values (Royal Commission on Aboriginal Peoples, 1996; Truth and Reconciliation Commission, 2015a, 2015b) driven by profit and self-interest. The Indian Residential School system, which operated from 1879 to 1996, was a central intergenerational weapon to eradicate Indigenous Knowledge[1] as language, family, and community connections were destroyed over six consecutive generations (Royal Commission on Aboriginal Peoples, 1996; Truth and Reconciliation Commission, 2015a, 2015b).

Indigenous students, and all students in Canada, have historically experienced the null curriculum where there is an absence of representation and lack of honouring Indigenous languages and curricular material, Indigenous stories, and Indigenous teachers in schools. Colonial government policy and law opposed and undermined Indigenous community governance and social structures (Begaye, 2008; Turner, 2006). The realities of the original peoples of Turtle Island within the context of foreign power: language and thought have been invisible and historical truths suppressed (Battiste, 1998; Dion, 2009; Little Bear, 2009; Kanu, 2011; Simpson, 2014). In the field of education, and within the context of schools in particular, there is a historical lack of relationship, or "unconstructive silence" as Laprise (2014) describes it – an invisible barrier between educators and Indigenous students and the larger community, which manifests in social and political distance. There is currently a movement underway of critical awakening to the long, negative and hurtful relationship between Aboriginal[2] people and schooling, and actions are being taken to interrupt hegemony in the academic institutions with validation of Indigenous Knowledge within post-secondary education.

Indigenous people are in the process of a critical awakening to intergenerational trauma and the ongoing violence of colonization, healing,

DOI: 10.4324/9781003205296-12

cultural resurgence and Indigenous Knowledge mobilization. The profile of Indigenous peoples within the Canadian population has been raised in recent years through media coverage of political and social movements, global environmental concerns and raw stories of injustice, including stories related to the global COVID-19 pandemic, anti-racism, and the shocking revelation of 5,000 Indigenous children's unmarked residential school graves. Global leadership (United Nations Declaration on the Rights of Indigenous Peoples, 2008), and national government (Truth and Reconciliation Commission of Canada 2015a, 2015b) and provincial responses and policies (Alberta Education, 2020a; Alberta Education, 2020b) illustrate a climate of change towards truth and reconciliation. Canada's Truth and Reconciliation Commission's (TRC's) Calls to Action (2015) have shaped the recently revised Alberta Education (2020a) *Teaching Quality Standard*, which now includes teaching competency no. 5: "A teacher develops and applies foundational knowledge about First Nations, Métis and Inuit for the benefit of all students" (p. 6). According to the Alberta Education (2020b) *Leadership Quality Standard*, school jurisdiction leaders are to support the application of foundational knowledge about First Nations, Métis, and Inuit.

With the advent of calls for educational reform in Canada, combined with a movement towards decolonization and social justice through critical theory, recent education policies and curricula revisions point to a variety of transformative possibilities. History is being redefined as Indigenous people tell their stories, and the crucial role for Indigenous Elders and critically aware educators (allies and Indigenous Teachers) within the classroom have come to light. An ally is a non-Aboriginal person in a "meaningful, non-oppressive" relationship of respect and trust with an Aboriginal person, which involves "a deep understanding of the interrelated and often mutually reinforcing complexities of power, privilege, identity, and difference" (Fitzmaurice, 2010, p. 364). Remembering Indigenous Knowledge and relational ways of knowing is relevant in contemporary education. Public schools are responsible for including Treaty education; the history and impacts of residential schools; and First Nations, Métis, and Inuit perspectives. The dawn of the new day for mutual respect and understanding creating integrative approaches for addressing issues and valuing different ways of knowing is upon us.

Following the release of the Truth and Reconciliation Commission of Canada's Calls to Action (TRC, 2015b), Canadian universities and colleges are responsible for indigenizing their institutions. There is opportunity to create space for Indigenous teaching-learning and cultural traditions and ethical Indigenous community-responsive research based on relationships. Based on a Canadian survey of 25 selected Indigenous and ally university academics, Gaudry and Lorenz (2018) identified a continuum of university indigenization efforts: at one end is Indigenous inclusion, with reconciliation indigenization in the centre, and decolonial indigenization at the other end, where "despite using a language of reconciliation, in practical terms the

Canadian academy still largely focuses on policies of inclusion. In contrast, Indigenous faculty, staff, students and their allies [envision a shift] based on principles of treaty and decolonial indigenization" (p. 226). It would seem a good place to meet could be in the middle at "reconciliation indigenization," which is one step closer to "decolonial indigenization." In this spirit, our chapter awakens creativity and imagination for educators engaged in anti-oppressive and Indigenous education by sharing stories and reflections in relation to a university research project titled "Growing Faculty, Staff and Student Foundational Knowledge of Indigenous Philosophies, Epistemologies, Ontologies, and Pedagogies."

The impetus for this book chapter arose from one co-researcher's interest in representing Indigenous women's voices in the knowledge dissemination aspect of the project. Originally, there were four women willing to share their stories in this chapter; however, the writing process took us on a journey of remembering traumas and tears and required lengthy discussions and deep thinking for critical reflections. As a result of this conscientious process, two women withdrew. The co-authors of this chapter have knowledge from lived experience with Indigenous healing, self-care, and wellness practices (in the project and beyond), and each time we gathered to reflect and write, we checked in with each other about how we were feeling, to share about our memories, and together we shed tears and many laughs. Spending time in nature, with Lands and Waters and sitting next to a gentle fire were effective strategies for rebalancing in this process.

Project Overview

In 2018, with provincial education funding, the Elementary Education Department, University of Alberta, embarked on the three-year exploratory research project titled "Growing Faculty, Staff and Student Foundational Knowledge of Indigenous Philosophies, Epistemologies, Ontologies, and Pedagogies." With a lens towards teaching innovation, the project endeavoured to enhance teacher education so that educators develop and apply foundational knowledge about First Nations, Métis, and Inuit for the benefit of all students (Alberta Education, 2020a). The broad research questions leading the project included: What are the elements of foundational Indigenous Knowledge? What principles and concepts are made visible in a Teaching Lodge? Specifically, how is *Anishinaabe* Knowledge socially enacted in the cultural traditions of teaching and learning? How does the co-researcher's engagement with Indigenous Knowledge and ways of teaching and learning transform their learning and educational praxis?

Twenty-five co-researchers in the undergraduate and graduate programmes at the University of Alberta, including the two Indigenous women who are the authors of this chapter, engaged in the project for three years. Participants were invited by members of the project initiators' group with purposeful recruitment of faculty members, graduate and undergraduate students (pre-service and in-service teachers), and faculty student service staff. Participants were co-researchers, documenting their own learning journeys with photographs, drawings, poetry, art, and written reflections. One-quarter of the participants were male and a wide range of ages was represented. The project Elder (male) had been involved with the group in a preliminary project and was selected with continuity of relationships in mind. Participants were inspirationally resilient, taking on the role of teachers in the education of the heart as well as the mind.

Tears of pain and anguish were shed in the project Teaching Lodge with personal stories of wounds from the systemic oppression of the university – harm associated with negative stereotypes and social attitudes that fuel racist and gendered violence. Stories shared and the retelling of stories contribute to knowledge transmission and new knowledge generation. Our decolonized Indigenous approach to storytelling involved centring ourselves as wholistic beings, including nurturing all aspects of ourselves (visioning/intuitive, doing, feeling/relating, and thinking) and engaging in ceremony in which our visions, dreams, and emotions were honoured.

Odawa Elder Stan Peltier, from *Wiikwemkoong* Unceded Territory, Ontario, provided guidance and Teachings, including bringing us into ceremony in the Teaching Lodge/tipi, which was set in a wooded area on a private acreage off campus. We focused on our collective journey of creating respectful and ethical relationships while engaging in a self-actualizing journey towards the acquisition of *Nibwakaawin*/Wisdom: "Life is like learning from everything that surrounds you and if you sort things out yourself, you become very intelligent. Your final goal with the Teachings is *Nibwakaawin/* Wisdom" (Stan Peltier, personal communication, 2018). Each Lodge began with a Teaching from Elder Stan, who encouraged us to consider how our experiences lived within the Lodge intersected with our personal lives and lives within the academy. Our relational Lodge pedagogy involved sharing, listening, and learning from each other's stories, and engaging our mental, emotional, spiritual, and physical ways of Being. For the two authors of this chapter, the Lodge was also a place of reclaiming our learning, for it allowed us the opportunity to learn the ways of our people and our ancestors that were otherwise denied through formal education, colonialism, language and territory loss, and other traumatic experiences. Our ancestors intended that we share who we are, our ways of knowing and being as Indigenous peoples, and live as equals with all other peoples in Canada. The ceremony of Circle provided a safe community context conducive to bringing our hearts and heads together.

Part of this reclaiming of our learning meant that the female pre-service teacher who is a co-author of this chapter, as well as other project helpers, were guided by Auntie Sharla. The young women learned how to speak words of gratitude and to sing for the *Odewiminan*/Strawberries and *Nibi/* Water. Elder Stan led the men to build and attend to the central fire. Both learned how to set the Lodge/tipi, and gradually, over time, adjustments to the smoke flaps and tipi liner were made so that the prevailing winds did not blow the smoke into our space (Figure 9.1).

A ceremonial Circle process of listening to stories and sharing stories allowed each individual to make meaningful connections. Long after the Circle had ended and the Teaching Lodge fire had died down, the stories stimulated deep knowing through a reflective process of remembering, relating, and wondering. In addition to the Teaching Lodge ceremonial gatherings, participants, as co-researchers, gathered round a praxis table to talk about reflections and new insights, and to share how new knowledge was being lived. Anecdotes of applications to curriculum, pedagogy, and student and faculty services in the university came to light.

Centring ourselves as wholistic Beings brings attention and nurturing to all aspects of ourselves (visioning/intuitive, doing, feeling/relating, and thinking), and in ceremony our visions, dreams, and emotions are honoured. The Teaching Lodge context was especially important to support us collectively and individually in our journey of storying and learning, and was essential in the process of unlearning what the colonial narrative has led us to internalize and believe about our ways of Being. Telling our stories

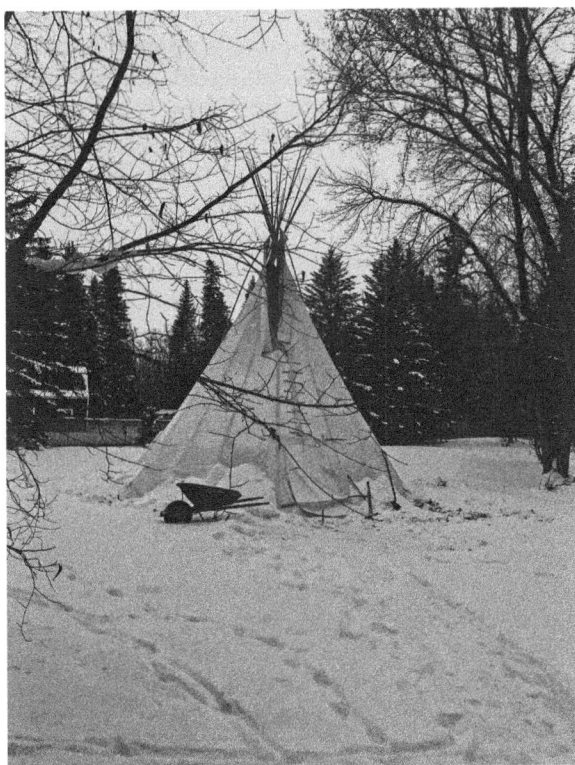

Figure 9.1 Teaching Lodge with Central Fire. Courtesy of Sharla Mskokii Peltier.

in a space of safety and equality brought us together as a collective with humility and empathy. We found a strong place of belonging. Our tears of pain and anguish are healing tears – part of our process of critical awakening and dedication to actions for positive transformation of the academy and education.

The stories that follow are reflections by two project participants that serve as counternarratives, bringing Indigenous Story Method into practice in academia. The power of story facilitates deeper learning through reflexivity. Through story, experiential knowledge is centred pushing back on colonial ways of knowing and being, making way for the knowledge and humanity of Indigenous peoples, which are centred in ceremony to lift up our spiritual and visioning wisdom. We invite readers to think with our stories and to be inspired towards personal possibilities of praxis for educational transformation by returning to reflect on the stories after reading the chapter, which also includes discussions related to theory and method, in addition to some final thoughts on moving forward on the path to reconciliation in education.

Resurgence of traditional values and ways of coming to know are the means towards rebuilding Indigenous identity and Wisdom, and strengthening family and community relationships. Each individual is situated within the centre of the Medicine Circle. There are four aspects to our being: visioning/spiritual, making/doing, relating/feeling, and thinking/knowing (Bopp et al., 1989). We seek harmony and balance within the wheel as we relearn our history and traditions that underlie our meaning and direction. Awaitka (1993) describes the process of "restoring harmony from the inside out, and of extending that concept from the individual to the community."(p. 283) It is in this spirit that we present our stories in this chapter. We are responsible for our own learning journey and are compelled to pass on the knowledge. In spite of the social and political contexts that do us harm, we strive to regain balance, do our healing work, and experience a sense of personal wellness. The relational and interdependent contexts of life lived means that wellness extends from us personally, moving outward in all directions, restoring positive energy and balance in our family, community, nation, and cosmology.

Charis's Story

Charis situates herself in relation to co-writing this chapter and her engagement in the project: I am a Two-Spirit Nêhiyaw educator, researcher, and helper who was raised within an urban context. My paternal lineage stems from Chief Joseph Bigstone, while my maternal lineage stems from Chief Papaschase. I feel it is important to recentre myself this way in order to remember my responsibilities to my Ancestors, and those yet to come. I admit that I did not know of my Ancestors prior to entering the privileged landscape of academia. How was I supposed to know when, historically speaking, I am not even supposed to be here or know who I am because of the ongoing colonial project? My experiences within Western education are filled with trauma associated with oppression, and although I did not have the language at the time to explain how I was feeling, the visceral effects are still felt today.

On March 27, 2014, the final National TRC event was held in Amiskwacîwâskahikan. As an intergenerational survivor of the Indian Residential School system, this continues to be a pivotal moment in my healing, unlearning, and relearning journey. It was during this moment in time when all of the intergenerational trauma that I experienced during utero, childhood, adolescence, and adulthood amalgamated into one big interconnected spiral. This is when all of the theoretical knowledge that I was unlearning and relearning through my Native Studies degree intertwined with my own lived experience, therefore causing everything to finally *click*. During my experience within my first degree, I carried a lot of shame because I did not speak my language, nor did I have experience or knowledge of ceremony. I remember the day that I learned I am a "Bill C-31,"[3] and according to colonial constructions of "Indian-ness" I am not a Status Indian. I felt this as another layer of shame – I was not good enough to be a "real Indian" (Lawrence, 2004, p. 231). I carried anger towards *Nimosôm*/my grandfather who gave up his Treaty rights so he could consume firewater, thus becoming disenfranchised. I felt guilty for having judged him this way, and as I write this today, I feel compassion for *Nimosôm*. Now I understand that he was coping the only way he knew how to because of the trauma he carried. I need to remember that he lived during a time when being an Indian consisted of existing within the colonial boundaries that sever kinship ties. He was taught that he was a heathen and a savage and not to speak his language, which meant that *Nikâwiy*/my mother could not teach me something that she did not know herself. I forgive *Nimosôm* and *Nikâwiy* and myself for not knowing the things that were systematically taken away from us.

I entered this project at an important time in my second degree. This was a time in my life where I was beginning to question why I went back to school and why I would put myself through this again. My first degree took me twice the amount of time as a non-Indigenous person; I wondered if for non-Indigenous students, it was easier to read course content without being triggered all the time. My first degree took a significant amount of time to complete because it was the first time I was exposed to the realities of colonization and the intergenerational reverberations on successive generations of Indigenous people such as myself. Through this process, I came to understand more deeply what Anishinaabe scholar Young (2010) calls *intergenerational narrative reverberations*, which "include the loss of language, traditional cultural knowledge, and spiritual and relational practices, particularly family relationships" (p. 289). This brings to mind the insight that if colonization did not happen to my Ancestors, I would not have paid tuition to know who I am, where I come from, and how history affects who

I am as a Two-Spirit *Nêhiyaw*. I carried a lot of shame and anger from my first degree, and this subsequently carried over to my second degree where I felt yet another layer of shame. I wondered if I was "healed enough" to become a teacher. I recognized that the wounds from my first degree had not healed as much as I had hoped as I entered the secondary education programme. I remember the moment when I was sitting in class and realized that I would be required to teach a curriculum that was created by mostly white men who view society through a capitalistic and heteronormative lens. As I sat in discomfort with this reality, I wondered if anyone else in my class felt a similar tension. I had always wondered why I never knew who I was or where I came from, and in this moment, I realized the education system I was subjected to when growing up did not create space for my diverse identities to be represented. I wondered about how I was supposed to know something that was not taught to me, and about how my teachers were supposed to teach something that they were not taught how to teach.

I am grateful for the project and for our Lodge. A truly inclusive and safe space was created in order for me to arrive authentically as an entire-Being. Through this, I was able to unpack my anger, grief, and trauma from my undergraduate degrees. I arrived at our Lodge awake to the fact that the presence of Indigenous people in the project did not guarantee that it would in fact be a safe space for me as a Two-Spirit *Nêhiyaw*. When one of the project initiators reached out to invite me, I initially thought that I did not have anything to bring to the project because I did not consider myself a helper in the traditional way since I did not grow up in community. Through this project and through our Lodge, I have been made to feel whole again by reconnecting to the Land and Water and place in the Circle. Prior to being in our Lodge, I walked with my shoulders down. However, I now walk with dignity and with a humble purpose. I feel like I have gained my rites of passage through this experience, which has helped me remain true to who I am as a Two-Spirit *Nêhiyaw* and helper.

Sharla's Story

Sharla's story illuminates the past and her lived experiences of colonial harm in the academy. She begins by situating herself as an *Anishinaabe Kwe*/Ojibway woman, Auntie, a new Indigenous scholar in the Faculty of Education, University of Alberta, and one of five members of the project initiator group:

Our vision, alongside Elder Stan (my husband), inspired the research project proposal. We are in our third year of the project and are working to create a community of co-researchers as participants. I am grateful for the challenging journey from the borderlands of academia to a space within academia where I am in relationship with multiple epistemologies and methods, my home community, and the academic community. With a sense of responsibility to the next generations, I work in academia to stop the cycle of institutional harm so that Indigenous students have access to post-secondary education experiences that support them to thrive in their journey towards Wisdom, and to resist the perpetuation of ignorance fuelled by complacency. I am amazed at the opportunities that exist in the context of being in a Faculty of Education.

I describe my background to make clearer my connection to Lands and Waters, Indigenous ceremonial spaces and ways, the roles of *Wayskapeeyos/Oshkaabewisag*,[4] and to ethical engagements in relationship with Indigenous community systems and values. I have lived experience in First Nations contexts. In my place of origin, I am known as *Mskokii Kwe* or Red Earth woman, and I am a member of the Loon Clan. I was raised by my parents and paternal grandmother. My father was from Mnjikaning and my mother was from Golden Lake First Nation. My identity and self-development are grounded in *Odenang* or where the heart is – my home and community of origin, Mnjikaning. I grew up on the eastern shore of Lake Couchiching. My father taught me how to live with the lake in a respectful way so that we could harvest fish, eat, and make a living selling bait and guiding. The lake was our life. *Odenang* is the foundation for who I am and who I am becoming. I consider myself extremely lucky and am grateful to have learned about Indigenous community ways, ceremonies, and the roles of Elders as mentors to community helpers in Alberta and in Ontario over the years. I am an *Anishinaabemowin*-learner. My father and paternal grandmother were fluent speakers of *Anishinaabemowin* and due to the intergenerational trauma of residential school, they did not pass on the language within our family.

The all-too-common legacy of culture and language loss stems from a lived experience for several generations that lacked validation for the crucial impact of *Anishinaabemowin* on culture, thought, and the acquisition of Wisdom. Colonial violence has undermined Aboriginal ways of Being and promoted the belief that only English language and a formal education present opportunities for success in life. Indigenous Knowledge is vast and layered, with dedicated practices around Medicine, healing ceremonies, harvesting and preserving foods, and rites of passage to keep the community strong. *Wayskapeeyos/Oshkaabewisag* accept a humble role as helpers and prepare for the day when their Elder/teacher grants them the right to carry out particular aspects of men's work in ceremonial and community life.

My story describes challenges I experienced in the project as the result of colonial university approaches to research. My intention is to illustrate my work as an Indigenous scholar and the importance of being situated within an Indigenous research project community, which is necessary for disrupting the status quo. The University of Alberta Elder Protocol document (2012) describes the community-based Elder–helper mentorship process as follows:

> Most of our Aboriginal people who aspire to a particular specialty have
> worked with Elders for at least twenty years and more, much like an

apprentice. Aboriginal people in their thirties, forties, and fifties, who work to serve their communities, work with Elders who have a particular specialty of interest to them: for example, Medicine People, or those who know how to conduct Pipe, Sweat Lodge, Sun Dance, Lodge, and other ceremonies, such as the Chicken Dance and the Horse Dance. Elders are recognized and identified by their respective communities according to the service they provide (p. 21)

Over the past four years I have been navigating the institutional structures of the university, in the process experiencing a myriad of difficult feelings and enduring a harsh process of becoming wakeful to many intriguing issues. In this chapter, I offer a few stories that illuminate the barriers I experienced and the disruption to my sense of well-being in my work as a project initiator in this research project. Policies and procedures perpetuate a Western colonial approach to education and research, and all-to-often the status quo overrides progress to shift relationships and university spaces based on principles of treaty and decolonial indigenization. Indigenous professors have been shaped by the academic landscape, which can be competitive and undermines a communal sense of solidarity in the advancement of reconciliation.

The project planning and early implementation phases were particularly challenging and stressful, yet our project initiator relationships and vision through ongoing discussions with participating Elder Stan Peltier saw the project through to fruition. To align with a relational curriculum and communal learning environment, Elder Stan and I visioned student participation in the project as helpers, which would support the movement underway in the urban Indigenous community that involves young Indigenous and Métis adults reconnecting with their people to continue their learning journey. We decided to seek one male and one female student as *Oshkaabewisag/Wayskapeeyos* who we would bring into the Teaching Lodge and support to learn protocols and take on the role of helpers at gatherings. We would also introduce them to community ceremonies and gatherings as a way of connecting to Indigenous communities by participating, observing, and offering to help. Over the course of the project, we mentored three male and two female *Oshkaabewisag/Wayskapeeyos*. These young people became an integral part of our Teaching Lodge and project activities, and established good relationships, which will continue to strengthen over time, with project co-participants and project initiators. We introduced the helpers to community members and Elders at powwows, Round Dances, Horse Dances, Winter Giveaway Ceremonies, and Tea Dances, which, in addition to the other project activities, contributed to the helpers gaining a sense of belonging, knowledge of community ways and protocols, and confidence to participate.

When I embarked on this research project journey, I had no idea how difficult it would be. For example, Alberta Education policies and procedures provided for appropriate compensation when engaging Indigenous community members and Elders in educational activities, and these principles were reflected in our project budget. Yet, our proposal came under scrutiny by officials with Western research lenses who questioned the proposed amount for the Elder honoraria. In response, an addendum to the original proposal cited the University of Alberta Elder Protocol: "The person making the request is the one who determines the monetary value and the gifts presented. The amount given and the kinds of gifts given can be seen as indicators on how much value is assigned by, or gratitude felt by, the recipient for the help they have received" (University of Alberta 2012, p. 24). Thankfully the document, based on Indigenous community-engaged research with input from well-informed participants, was respected by ministry of education project reviewers and made a compelling case for our research budget.

I was naive and thought that policies and procedures would already be in place for Indigenous research in the Faculty of Education. As I tried to navigate the internal structures and financial, research system, I became extremely frustrated and felt like giving up so many times. The required Research Ethics Board clearance for our project took three months of tedious work to move the project forward. The research proposal described a participant researcher methodology where participants take on concurrent roles as research subjects and researchers, contributing their stories and artefacts of learning and praxis for knowledge dissemination. The research ethics application did not accommodate this approach and many questions were posed by reviewers.

In addition, the online research ethics application format did not accommodate Indigenous research methods and community-based approaches. For example, our approach was to gather information through Story Circles and to invite co-researchers to create their own representations of their learning and contributions to services and the university, to document the research project. The only category for data collection that seemed close to our method was "focus group" and we had no other option but to select this on the application form. In total, the research ethics application and review process generated 93 edits to our proposal! I was overwhelmed with the work involved and burden of making concise responses to maintain the integrity of engaging in Indigenous research methodology. Our project research initiators supported each other emotionally and shared the workload so that our project was eventually approved through research ethics.

When Western research ethics are applied in academic research, it becomes clear from my experiences at the university that Indigenous research is not well understood and Indigenous community ethics are questioned. In my experience as an *Anishinaabe Kwe* living in First Nations contexts, I have developed a good understanding of ethical community relational ways. I perceive my family and community within a broad kinship system. My relationships and knowledge of community resource people with capacity to support educational research projects in specific ways means that family members are involved. As a scholar engaged in Indigenous research, I understand my responsibilities and how to act with integrity and uphold ethical behaviour. I have a fluid and expansive sense of my family relationships which extend beyond blood relatives to encompass diverse relations including sisters, brothers, aunties, uncles, grandmothers, and grandfathers, in places on Turtle Island and beyond. The colonial power of the Indian Act established Reserves since the eighteenth and nineteenth centuries, and according to this, the First Nations context means living inside government-imposed borders. Within a First Nations context I am related by blood to most of the people in my community. A Western conception of family holds a nuclear perspective, with parents, children, and immediate family members who are blood relatives.

Western institutional policies are meant to ensure that a researcher does not engage in a conflict of interest within a capitalistic society where blood relatives are favoured to benefit directly from research project funds. From an Indigenous paradigm, Indigenous research projects engage the community and so from an Indigenous researcher perspective, it is inappropriate to exclude blood relatives or people considered to be family. My role as a project initiator includes budget management, and a collision of Western and Indigenous ideologies and ethics resulted in my integrity being questioned by faculty administrators regarding this project. When foreign values are applied and scrutiny occurs, my integrity as an Indigenous researcher and faculty member and my reputation are harmed. I experience being disrespected and my feelings of self-doubt and pain take a toll on me. Many tears were shed and I managed to rise to the challenge by refusing to participate in the harm. I did not agree to sign a conflict-of-interest statement. I am grateful that project initiators supported me with a letter explaining the relationships and absence of conflicting interests.

As I reflect on my experiences navigating the institutional structures of the university through this project, I once again experience feelings of shame and hurt. The central fire in the Lodge has provided a much-needed safe place to notice my feelings and thoughts, and to create a Circle of storytellers with hearts and heads together. This has brought healing and movement towards positive change. Although I revisit negative experiences and feelings in this writing, I also acknowledge and feel gratitude for the project initiators and participant co-researchers. Shedding tears and sharing stories brings forward an empathetic community awake to the harm that colonial institutions such as the university continue to inflict on Indigenous people. A sense of solidarity within this writing group brings strength to name the oppressive colonial narratives and institutional structures, and to refuse to live within a violent system in silence.

Indigenous Knowledge as Experience, Oral Tradition, and Indigenous Knowledge Transmission

Indigenous Knowledge is transmitted through Indigenous language, experiential learning, ceremony, and intergenerational learning. Scholars from diverse academic and cultural perspectives have provided information about Indigenous Knowledge as a process situated within a context of relationships. Indigenous Knowledge is rooted in Place and community, and is an animated process and experience. Indigenous people are diverse. Each cultural community possesses its own language and has a system of beliefs and values based on experience, which are articulated in the philosophy of the oral tradition. Cree philosopher Willie Ermine (1995) discusses Indigenous Knowledge as an interaction of life experience, relational collectivity, and inner knowing (p. 104). Each of us is situated in a specific place and Indigenous Knowledge is a way of Being, knowing, and doing – a lifelong process that involves observing, listening, engaging in life activities, and developing skills modelled by family and community members.

Indigenous Knowledge is inherently tied to a web of relationships. Ceremonies provide complete and accurate transmission of knowledge and authority from generation to generation. Battiste (2002) identifies the learning process of ceremony as modelling customs for acquiring and sharing knowledge, competent and respectful behaviour, and demonstrating spirit-connecting processes enabling the learner's unique gifts (inherent talents and capabilities), vision, and spirit to emerge. Learning is self-directed with knowledge gained from introspection, reflection, meditation, and prayer. The learner comes to know their own gifts and capabilities, strengths and weaknesses, interests, and limits to develop self-knowledge and esteem. Ceremonies support understanding of relationships and values reflected in Indigenous language. Connecting with Wisdom and traditions of Indigenous Knowledge nurtures all aspects of the learner in a harmonious way, while Western knowledges and pedagogical traditions privilege written word and cognitive processes. An Indigenous learner experiences fragmentation and disconnection in school where the dominant idea of deficit thinking is directed towards Indigenous learners and Indigenous ways of knowing are subordinate to dominant ways of knowing. The Indigenous learner's living process of knowledge is subjugated by colonial power, generation upon generation.

Indigenous Knowledge and cultural Teachings in the form of oral traditions have been handed down by the Elders to the young for centuries. According to Kulnieks et al. (2010), in addition to being deeply connected to place, "traditional stories from Indigenous elders [keep] an interconnected body of ancestral knowledge alive" (p. 20), which is an important motivating factor for younger generations to contribute to the longevity of their traditions. Indigenous orality encompasses oratory skills for leadership, transmitting history, and in storytelling, which reflects Truth and walking in two worlds or seeing physical and spiritual life. What a person shares from the heart is considered to be their truth. Indigenous Knowledge requires a reflective process of deep meaning-making so that our stories and oral tradition stimulate remembering; when we retell stories, we contribute to knowledge transmission and new knowledge generation.

Indigenous philosophy and ways of knowing are part of a wholistic, generative process that is inextricably tied to ancient language. The contributions of *Anishinaabemowin*[5] and *Nêhiyawewin*/Cree language by project participants convey worldview perspectives and exemplify Indigenous ways of knowing. Incorporating Indigenous languages in our Teaching Lodges and project initiation work has been key to our teaching-learning process and decolonizing indigenization work.

Indigenous Story Method

This chapter includes reflective writing by two Indigenous women and provides insights on storying and deep knowing within ceremonial and narrative ways. This contributes to a vision for healing and educational praxis through an Indigenous Story Method (Kovach, 2009; Wilde, 2003). Experiences and coming to know from a relational way of being characterize Indigenous Knowledge, which is a form of *Debwewin*, the *Anishinaabemowin* term for Truth rooted in one's heart (Gehl, 2012). Our work as Indigenous women is informed by critical Indigenous theory, which draws attention to the need to balance power relations in the academy and to resist cultural hegemony. Indigenous inquiry is also about giving back to individual and collective good where "[r]esearch in service of social and ecological justice is inseparable from this value" (Kovach, 2009, p. 174).

An Indigenous paradigm supports this relational, participants-as-researchers method, and involves respect for the topic and being sensitive to people's feelings about research outcomes. As Indigenous women storytellers, we were conscious that our individual stories had power to transform spaces and places. The stories we share are our Truth and we take on the responsibility for passing on the knowledge with respect for Lodge participants and readers of this chapter. As we shared stories in the Teaching Lodge, we contributed to the naming of oppression. Each Story Circle in the Lodge began with the provocation, "What have you been thinking about and doing in your educational work since our last gathering?" This open invitation to share in the Lodge, where equality and respect were centred, meant that participants shared their truth without feeling guarded about their story. The Lodge Circle process of listening, sharing stories, and ceremony raised consciousness. Ceremony brought faculty, students, and staff together within an Indigenous paradigm of sacred ethical space to gather in humble reverence of our place in cosmology alongside our ancestors. A ceremonial Circle process of listening to stories and sharing stories allowed each individual to make meaningful connections. Long after the Circle had ended and the Teaching Lodge fire extinguished, shared stories stimulated deep knowing through the reflective process of remembering, relating, and wondering.

The Indigenous Story Method was also applied at the praxis table, where co-researchers were invited to share tea and participate in a Story Circle to explore one of our most important research questions: How does the co-researcher's engagement with Indigenous Knowledge and ways of teaching and learning transform their learning and educational praxis? Each gathering began with participants sharing experiences and reflections on the Teaching Lodge. Gatherings were recorded, transcribed, and included in project reports. Transcriptions were shared electronically with those in attendance. These included reflections, shared insights, and stories about how new knowledge was being lived, including anecdotes related to curriculum, pedagogy, and student and faculty services.

Ceremony as Ethical Space

Educational transformation calls us to work within ethical space. In our exploratory research, the ceremonial Teaching Lodge provided a framework and Place of sacred ethical space. The significance of spirituality and ceremony in lifelong learning for Indigenous people is great. Elder Yvonne Vizina expressed the sentiment that spiritual experiences are integral to each person's learning journey, and are honoured through ceremony and relationships with the community's spiritual leaders (Canadian Council on Learning, 2008) (Figure 9.2).

If the university is to exude a reconciliatory environment, it is necessary to disrupt Western conceptions of knowledge and hierarchy in the learner–teacher relationship. The framework of ethical space presents opportunities for Western and Indigenous ethical/moral principles to co-exist in cross-cultural cooperation. Willie Ermine describes the condition for ethical space as being an affirmation of human diversity created by philosophical and cultural differences. A neutral zone for a meeting between cultures with contrasting perspectives of the world ensues in an ideological theatre for cross-cultural conversation in pursuit of ethically engaging diversity. Ermine (2007) envisions this "new partnership model of the ethical space, in a cooperative spirit between Indigenous peoples and Western institutions [to] create new currents of thought that flow in different directions and overrun the old ways of thinking" (p. 203).

Circles during ceremonies in the Lodge were a safe and sacred space where people were encouraged to share, and listeners did not disclose details outside the Lodge. Definitions and boundaries of what is considered professional or appropriate in the academy are left behind and instead humans can be vulnerable and share their emotional, mental, and spiritual selves. This abandonment for what is considered a professional demeanour allows Lodge participants to connect through true and honest expression of what it means to be a human within their personal lives and within the academy. The lodge facilitates connection, empathy, and equality where everyone has an equal voice. It is through this accepting and loving environment that people are willing to share personal stories of their families, lives, schooling, and the academy. The safety of the Lodge allowed people

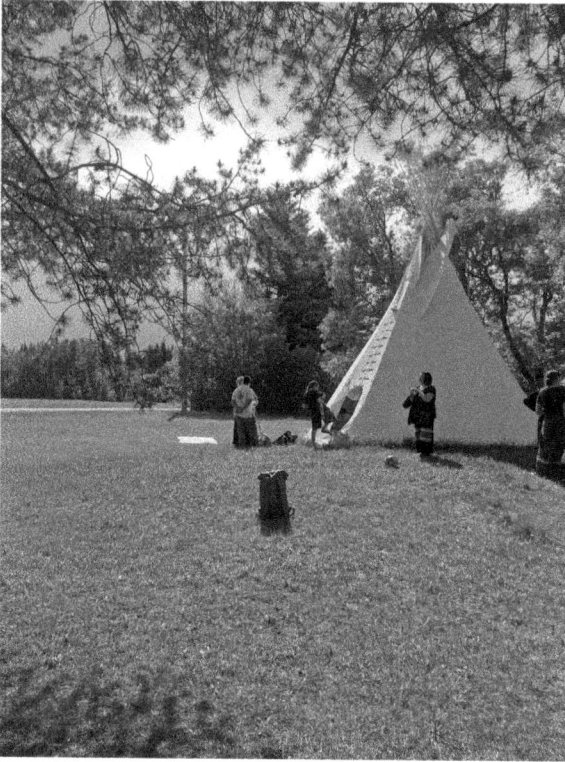

Figure 9.2 Project participants gathering at Teaching Lodge. Courtesy of Sharla
Mskokii Peltier.

to share their stories of pain and fear, and experiences of judgement and
interpersonal violence. As Indigenous women, we cried together as a means
of healing together. Shedding tears as a ceremony of healing reflects a pedagogy of engaging with pain and suffering, which honours the words of survivor Evelyn Brockwood, who expressed the importance of slowing down
so that all people affected by residential schools take the time for healing
to occur: "We have many tears to shed before we even get to the word
reconciliation" (TRC Final Report, 2015a, p. 11). We were motivated by
"auntie" Evelyn's wisdom to slow down our living in these times of truth-
telling and healing.

Moving Forward

Canadian social and academic spheres have been positively impacted by the
work of critical Indigenous scholars, educators, and political leaders who
are cognizant of the historical colonialist dialogue concerning Indigenous

education and who have made a call for educational transformation. Indigenous scholars and students continue to find themselves enmeshed in educational institution processes that reflect colonial approaches to policy in terms of privileging Western ways, thus creating barriers for them. One example is standards for recognition of knowledge, which do not typically include a recognized Indigenous form of knowledge derived from attending to the Learning Spirit and feelings.

We see the benefit of slowing down so that we engage in purposeful truth-telling, critical thinking, and reflections for deeper understanding and attending to all aspects of ourselves to nurture emotional and spiritual well-being. With healing comes visioning and engagement in reconciliation that comes from agency in actions for transformative change in the academy. We shared stories of lived experience and our journeys of awakening with respect to how we were harmed by institutional oppression and systemic racism. We unapologetically expressed our feelings and vulnerabilities to connect as human beings. Our sense of solidarity brought much strength to naming oppression and framing accountability. We are accountable to continue the work of learning, unlearning, and disrupting the normalizing colonial practices that cause harm in education.

With respect to our "Growing Faculty, Staff and Student Foundational Knowledge of Indigenous Philosophies, Epistemologies, Ontologies, and Pedagogies" research project, participants' experiences, reflections, and a process of critical awakening have unfolded to inform the praxis students, staff, faculty, and department staff and administrators towards enhancement of the teacher education programme and advancement of decolonial indigenization. The collective experiences of project participants from experiencing and reflecting on a wholistic relational pedagogy have led to the creation of Indigenous ethical spaces such as storytelling Circles and ceremonies, and gradual changes to research approaches so that Indigenous and relational pedagogies and curriculum making are being brought forward into university spaces. A shift in methodology towards a pedagogy that allows us to be relational beings while creating ethical and decolonial spaces within the academy is a taking back of our spirits and power as Indigenous Peoples (Episkenew, 2009; Palmater, 2017).

Engagement with decolonial indigenization is emancipatory work from the margins that aligns with the movement of anti-oppressive education. Brown and Strega (2005) describe motivation "to make space and take space for marginalized researchers and ideas" (p. 2). Through this project, we have gained further lived experience in the challenging work of bringing our heads and hearts together to empower each other and resist as a community. As individuals, today we feel a sense of power and assertiveness. Our project and its collective processes brought change to our lives as we moved from the margins to the Circle of belonging around the central fire in the Teaching Lodge and at praxis table gatherings. We share our experiences as insights for a way forward to guide and inspire others working in university contexts. The difficult and overwhelming work of decolonial indigenization is long term, as change does not happen right away.

During our current post-TRC context in Canada, more academic institutions are being populated by Indigenous people. Indigenous people hold the key and may extend an invitation for others to join the Circle of ethical space so that eventually, Indigenous languages, Indigenous Knowledge, ways of researching and coming to know, and traditions of teaching-learning will have a welcomed place in the university. We invite readers of this chapter to think with our stories and be inspired towards personal possibilities of praxis for educational transformation. A ceremonial Teaching Lodge is a structural change in the Western academy. The ethical space of a central fire and ceremony is a wonderful environment necessary for creating relationships of mutual respect and understanding among Indigenous and non-Indigenous faculty, students, and staff. In the Lodge, feelings and lived experience, and stories of anger, grief, shame, guilt, and denial are powerfully mobilized to facilitate a shift to wakefulness and altered worldviews.

We honour the important principle of non-interference. We are not responsible for your journey and we do not overstep by instructing others on what they should do. We give away our stories to inspire and guide you as you engage in meaning-making. You have the capacity to think critically, to reflect, and to decide on actions that resonate with you and your Learning Spirit. Wakefulness and attendance to personal healing work will lend strength to capacity-building and collaboration, thereby dismantling the status quo. Safe journey.

Acknowledgement

We wish to acknowledge and thank Dr. Stephanie Pyne, Ottawa, Ontario, for her "deep editing" services, kindness, and care for our manuscript.

Notes

1 The textual style for Indigenous language terms and other concepts (Land, Elders) are capitalized in this chapter to reflect the importance of these terms in this research paradigm.
2 The term *Aboriginal* is commonly used in Canada and is used here to refer specifically to the Indigenous people in Canada (Helin, 2006). *Aboriginal* is the word used in Canada's Constitution and includes "Indians, Inuit and Métis."
3 "Bill C-31, or a Bill to Amend the Indian Act, passed into law in April 1985 to bring the Indian Act into line with gender equality under the Canadian Charter of Rights and Freedoms" (Indigenous Foundations, 2009).
4 *Wayskapeeyos* is a Nêhiyaw/Cree language term and *Oshkaabewisag* is an Anishinaabemowin term to describe those who work as helpers alongside Elders and ceremonialists at gatherings.
5 *Anishinaabemowin* refers to the Aboriginal languages of the Anishinaabek people, spoken by the Algonquin, Chippewa, Delaware, Mississauga, Odawa, and Ojibway and Pottawatomi people of the Great Lakes Region. The language used

throughout this chapter comes from Elder Stan's teachings of *Anishinaabemowin* concepts and principles that are foundational to Indigenous thinking and ways of knowing.

References

Alberta Education. (2020a). *Teaching quality standard*. Retrieved from https://open .alberta.ca/dataset/4596e0e5-bcad-4e93-a1fb-dad8e2b800d6/resource/75e96af5 -8fad-4807-b99a-f12e26d15d9f/download/edc-alberta-education-teaching -quality-standard-2018-01-17.pdf

Alberta Education. (2020b). *Leadership quality standard*. Retrieved from https:// open.alberta.ca/dataset/b49851f6-d914-4f28-b5d5-199b028beeca/resourhenry ce/cf0fede2-3895-4ed5-a2d9-23610dccb2d9/download/edc-leadership-quality -standard-english-2020.pdf

Awaitka, M. (1993). *Selu: Seeking the corn-mother's wisdom*. Fulcrum Publishing.

Battiste, M. (1998). Enabling the autumn seed: Toward a decolonized approach to aboriginal knowledge, language, and education. *Canadian Journal of Native Education, 22*, 16–28.

Battiste, M. (2002). *Indigenous knowledge and pedagogy in first nations education: A literature review with recommendations* (p. 69). National Working Group on Education, INAC.

Begaye, T. (2008). Modern democracy: the complexities behind appropriating indigenous models of governance and implementation. In Handbook of critical and indigenous methodologies (pp. 459–470). SAGE Publications, Inc., https:// dx.doi.org/10.4135/9781483385686

Bopp, J., Bopp, M., Brown, L., & Lane, P. (1989). *The sacred tree*. Lotus Press.

Brown, L., & Strega, S. (2005). Introduction: Transgressive possibilities. In L. Brown & S. Strega (Eds.), *Research as resistance: Critical indigenous and anti-oppressive approaches* (pp. 1–17). Canadian Scholars Press.

Canadian Council on Learning. (2008). *Nourishing the learning spirit: Elder's dialogue*. Aboriginal Learning Knowledge Centre.

Dion, S. (2009). *Braiding histories: Learning from aboriginal peoples' experiences and perspectives*. UBC Press.

Episkenew, J. A. (2009). *Taking back our spirits: Indigenous literature, public policy, and healing*. University of Manitoba Press.

Ermine, W. (1995). Aboriginal epistemology. In M. Battiste & J. Barman (Eds.), *First nations education in Canada: The circle unfolds* (pp. 101–112). UBC Press.

Ermine, W. (2007). The ethical space of engagement. *Indigenous Law Journal, 6*(1), 193–203.

Gaudry, A., & Lorenz, D. (2018). Indigenization as inclusion, reconciliation, and decolonization: Navigating the different visions for indigenizing the Canadian academy. *AlterNative, 14*(3), 218–227.

Gehl, L. (2012). Debwewin journey: A methodology and model of knowing. *AlterNative: An International Journal of Indigenous Peoples, 8*(1), 53–65.

Helin, C. (2006). *Dances with dependency*. Orca Spirit Publishing and Communications, Inc.

Henderson, J. Y. (2012). Post-colonial ghost dancing: Diagnosing European colonialism. In M. Battiste (Ed.), *Reclaiming indigenous voice and vision* (pp. 57–76). UBC Press.

Kanu, Y. (2011). *Integrating aboriginal perspectives into the school curriculum: Purposes, possibilities, and challenges*. University of Toronto Press.

Kovach, M. (2009). *Indigenous methodologies: Characteristics, conversations, and contexts*. University of Toronto Press.

Kulnieks, A., Longboat, D. R., Young, K. (2010). Re-indigenizing curriculum: An eco-hermeneutic approach to learning. *AlterNative: An International Journal of Indigenous Scholarship*, 6(1), 15–24.

Laprise, M. (2014). Freedom of knowledge: Why the incorporation of aboriginal perspectives in Canadian education systems is vital. *Undergraduate Journal of Indigenous Studies/Dbaajimowin*, 2, 123–132.

Lawrence, B. (2004). *"Real" Indians and others: Mixed-blood urban native peoples and indigenous nationhood*. University of Nebraska Press.

Little Bear, L. (2009). *Naturalizing indigenous knowledge, synthesis paper*. Aboriginal Learning Knowledge Centre – Canadian Council on Learning Retrieved from NaturalizingIndigenousKnowledge_LeroyLittlebear.pdf (neatoeco.com)

Palmater, P. (2017). Decolonizing is taking back our power. In P. McFarlane & N. Schabus (Eds.), *Whose land is it anyway? A manual for decolonization* (pp. 73–78). Federation of Post-Secondary Educators of BC. https://fpse.ca/sites/default/files/news_files/Decolonization%20Handbook.pdf

Royal Commission on Aboriginal Peoples. (1996). *Report of the Royal Commission on aboriginal peoples*. Canada Communications Group.

Simpson, L. (2014). Land as pedagogy: Nishinaabeg intelligence and rebellious transformation. Decolonization: Indigeneity, Education & Society, 3(3), 1–25. Retrieved from http://decolonization.org/index.php/des/article/view/22170/17985

Truth and Reconciliation Commission. (2015a). *Truth and Reconciliation Commission of Canada: Calls to action*. Retrieved from http://trc.ca/assets/pdf/Calls_to_Action_English2.pdf

Truth and Reconciliation Commission of Canada. (2015b). *Canada's residential schools: Reconciliation. The final report of the Truth and Reconciliation Commission of Canada, Volume 6*. Retrieved from http://www.trc.ca/assets/pdf/Volume_6_Reconciliation_English_Web.pdf

Turner, D. (2006). This is not a piece pipe: Towards a critical *indigenous* philosophy. University of Toronto Press.

United Nations Declaration on the Rights of Indigenous Peoples (2008). *United nations general assembly resolution 61/295, September*. Retrieved from http://www.un.org/esa/socdev/unpfii/documents/DRIPS_en.pdf

University of Alberta. (2012). Elder protocol (Council on Aboriginal Initiatives, February 11, 2012). Retrieved from https://cloudfront.ualberta.ca/-/media/ualberta/office-of-the-provost-and-vice-president/indigenous-files/elderprotocol.pdf

Wilde, K. (2003). Storytelling as a methodology. In J. Oakes, R. Riewe, A. Dubois, A. Edmunds, & K. Wilde (Eds.), *Native voices in research* (pp. 191–198). University of Manitoba, Aboriginal issues press.

Young, M., Chester, J.-L., Flett, B. M., Joe, L., Marshall, L., Moore, D., Paul, K., Paynter, F., Williams, J., & Huber, J. (2010). Becoming "real" aboriginal teachers: Attending to intergenerational narrative reverberations and responsibilities. *Teachers and Teaching*, 16(3), 285–305. Retrieved from https://doi-org.login.ezproxy.library.ualberta.ca/10.1080/13540601003634370

10 Remembering Other Ways to Live

The Healing Energy that Flows from Sacred Ecology

Zahra Kasamali

Introduction

This chapter is inspired by what was missing from my own education on formal schooling landscapes and my continued commitments to expanding the practice of anti-racism through direction from wisdom-guided sacred ecological philosophies (Cardinal & Hildebrandt, 2000; Dei, 1996; Donald, 2019; Kasamali, 2020; Kasamali, 2021; Kumashiro, 2004; Morris, 2002). My K–12 schooling experiences revealed the extent to which curricular outcomes and pedagogical practices had become reliant on approaches to difference that were mired in colonial logics and dependent on the false universalism of liberalism. Following Paine (1999), Turner (2006), and Venn (2002), I conceptualize the false universalism of liberal philosophy as the currency of liberal ideological structures in institutional spaces that normalize the rhetoric of sameness through difference. Conceptions of cosmopolitan communities within the Enlightenment period explicate the origins of sameness through difference and deny other ways of living that called into question the dominance of the liberal Canadian nation-state. My location and positionality as a Pakistani-Canadian Muslimah (Muslim woman), who was raised within Sufic traditions in Islam and raised in Alberta, gifted me with the opportunity to ethically enact the place-based knowledges and philosophies of Treaty 6 territory, and the holistic message of Islam with balance and integrity. The sadness and anxieties that resulted from continuously being storied as a problem, especially for my Muslimness, gave rise to years of separating myself from my embodied knowledges, distance from the wisdom of Islam and its guidance on institutional landscapes, and forgetting my relationship with my more-than-human relatives. These experiences and complex emotions were exacerbated by the tragic events of September 11, 2001. Widely known as 9/11, it refers to four coordinated attacks that took place in New York City; Arlington, Virginia; and near Washington DC. Monolithic reports of 9/11 have narrativized the instigators of this event as "Islamic terrorists" or fundamentalists (Kasamali, 2021). Following 9/11, I found myself continuously forced to apologize for these acts, and defending the integrity of one billion Muslims globally.

DOI: 10.4324/9781003205296-13

Such impositions accelerated the self-hatred I internalized and manifested unhealthy reactions to Islamophobia. These struggles distanced me from Islam's life-giving energy that I needed to connect with in order to walk in good ways alongside all living beings. At this time, my mental, emotional, physical, and spiritual solace was limited to family members, and I was being uplifted by community gatherings and prayers.

Consequently, I explored the curricular and pedagogical significance of holism in deepening understandings of difference. This research was inspired by my former experiences as a committed critical theorist who heavily relied upon anti-racist pedagogy to support marginalized students in a high school context with a large population of recent newcomers and First Nations, Métis, and Inuit students. My teaching experiences called into question the efficacy of anti-racism to support healing from traumatic lived experiences on curricular and pedagogical sites. I was astounded that students with whom I had established a relationship were not connecting with anti-racism in the ways that I assumed they would, and in the ways that the research indicated. These happenings, along with witnessing how students at times felt critical theory practices were too prescriptive, assumptive, and imposing (Ellsworth, 1989), convinced me to address what I had overlooked. My doctoral study opened up how holistic sensibilities can support healing, balance, and kinship on schooling sites when youth are given opportunities to reconnect with sacred ecology (Kasamali, 2019).

As a social studies and English language arts teacher working in an urban high school in Alberta, Canada, I was also gifted with the opportunity to learn from the curricular and pedagogical context of Aboriginal Studies 30. Aboriginal Studies 30 is a provincially mandated course in Alberta that is offered in senior high school at three levels. Alberta's provincial government is responsible for the curriculum that is disseminated to schools. The provincial curriculum provides a framework for what students are to learn and complete in subject areas and grade levels from kindergarten to grade 12. Aboriginal Studies 30 is guided by sacred ecological insights that promote and nurture living in balance and harmony. Sacred ecology refers to entities that make life possible, such as the sun, water, wind, and earth. Sacred ecology emphasizes that human beings and our more-than-human relational network (i.e. the four leggeds) are interconnected and dependent on each other for survival (Cardinal & Hildebrandt, 2000; Donald, 2019).

The etymology of *consciousness* explicates the term as "internal awareness" (and the "state of being aware of what passes in one's own mind") (Online Etymology Dictionary, 2021). The absence of cultivating "internal awareness" as integral to honouring historical consciousness is concerning because it closes off the generative potential of learning from embodied knowledges, kinship with human beings and our more-than-human relatives, and varied lived experiences and different ways of knowing and being. The genesis of an anthropocentric curriculum distances us from transformative sources of meaning-making and renewal. What is at stake in curricular and pedagogical practices that forget these relationships is the removal of a deepened connectivity that is needed to open up non-assimilatory expressions of difference that can guide living with greater integrity and balance. The absence of consciousness in deeper ways promotes imbalance of curricular and pedagogical landscapes because the erasure of generative experiences of difference makes people unwell (Some, 1994).

Given these tensions, it is essential to note that holism does not have a singular definition and is guided by different philosophies and practices. Holistic philosophies can be understood in connection to the plethora of global wisdom traditions that offer, in their own ways, contrasting ways to live wisely and well (Donald, 2009; Smith, 2006, 2014). Global wisdom traditions, while sharing certain common principles, espouse contrasting interpretations and are honoured and enacted in unique ways. It is also necessary to locate holistic sensibilities within the purview of religion and spirituality because many individuals conceptualize holism in this regard. Experiences and conceptualizations of religion and spirituality are also highly subjective and cannot be defined in monolithic ways (Zinnbauer et al., 1997). Therefore, this chapter is not seeking a cogent way to define holism or specific principles of holism; to do so would reduce the meaning of how individuals connect with these insights from their own sensibilities. I will, however, riff off the holistic insights of former Aboriginal Studies 30 student participants to assist with opening up these understandings and their utility in curricular and pedagogical contexts. My research inquiry is guided by the following question: *To what extent does the false universalism of liberalism reaffirm self-enclosed and intellectualized curricular and pedagogical approaches that miss notions of consciousness that promote connectivity with self, others, and nature?* In exploring this question, this chapter will illuminate the experiences of four former Aboriginal Studies 30 students – Alissa, Rose, Levi, and Chauntelle – and explore how sacred ecological philosophies can support healing on schooling landscapes.

This chapter is inspired by the wisdom-guided sacred ecological Cree philosophies of *miyo-wahkohtowin* (laws that govern good relationships) and *miyo-wîcêhtowin* (relationships of harmony) as sources of inspiration for life and living. Sufic philosophies, as espoused in Qur'anic teachings and Maulana Jalaluddin Rumi's poetry, explicate the concepts of *Tawhid*, *Ayat*, *Zahir* and *Batin*, and *Ashraf al-Makhluqat*. These teachings encourage the recovery of self and deepened expressions of connectivity that Canadian liberal multiculturalism cannot address. I will begin by unpacking sacred ecological teachings, as expressed in Qur'anic teachings related to Rumi's poetry. I seek inspiration from Rumi's poetry as I was born into a Sufic orientation in Islam and was frequently guided by Rumi's stories and poetry through family and community gatherings. The representation of Rumi's persona and teachings are far too often removed from Islam. For these reasons, amplifying Rumi's voice is a humble attempt to reclaim Qur'anic teachings that continue to be distorted and misunderstood. I will then provide a brief literature review that articulates shared Indigenous sacred ecological philosophies and then situate the Aboriginal Studies 30 experience by offering a philosophical overview of the course. Thirdly, I will share Alissa's, Rose's, Levi's, and Chauntelle's experiences with learning from the wisdom that flows from sacred ecology. Their individual and collective voices will be revealed through the métissage research sensibility. These insights will be interpreted through the hermeneutic interplay between former Aboriginal Studies 30 students' learnings from Cree philosophies, as inspired through the guidance of Elder Bob Cardinal from Enoch Cree Nation, Alberta, and Rumi's poems "One Task" and "The Truth Within Us." This hermeneutic interplay will aesthetically represent how healing from experiences of colonial exclusions is possible through reconnection with self and remembering and internalizing shared ecological philosophies on pedagogical landscapes. Lastly, these understandings will be further extrapolated through a curriculum discussion that evidences how opportunities to reconnect with self and kinship relational networks can inspire healing through learning to trust and seek guidance from the truths that exist within us all.

Qur'anic Teachings and Their Expression in Rumi's Poetry

The following section will specifically explore the Qur'anic teachings of *Tawhid*, *Zahir* and *Batin*, *Ayat*, and *Ashraf al-Makhluqat*. In North American contexts, Qur'anic teachings are far too often represented as rigid codified laws that are of little value to life and living, and removed from the deep reverence of Rumi's poetry. Pejorative representations of Islam and Muslims as violent individuals who practise an extremist faith and lifestyle continues to evoke fear and inexplicable hatred. Such assumptions have deleterious consequences on the ways in which many relate with Qur'anic wisdoms and Muslims. These teachings will also be explicated to help address their utility in curricular and pedagogical contexts as sources of guidance that can help restore balance.

Islam in general teaches the importance of living in balanced ways. The doctrine of *Tawhid*, or unity of all life forms, teaches that Allah created the universe in "perfect balance and measure" (Islamic Sciences and Research Academy Australia [ISRA], 2012, p. 11). The Qur'an and *Hadith* remind humankind that they ought not disrupt this balance (p. 11). The Qur'an states, "And the sky has raised high, and has devised (for all things) a balance, so that you might never transgress the balance: weigh, therefore, (your deeds), you with equity and do not upset the balance" (55:7–9). The Qur'an designates human beings as *Ashraf al-Makhluqat*, or the most noble of Creation. It is understood that Allah granted human beings, in *Amanah* (trust), the responsibility to maintain and strengthen Creation (ISRA, 2012, p. 17). Thus, human beings are entrusted to maintain the perfect balance that Allah created and to remember the practice of accountability.

The Qur'an emphasizes the inextricable relationship between *Zahir* and *Batin*, which sustains and strengthens this balance. *Zahir* is one of Allah's 99 names and represents the material, exoteric, and visible elements of life. In other words, *Zahir* is understood as form. *Batin* is also one of Allah's 99 names and corresponds to the spiritual, esoteric, and hidden. The teachings of balancing *Zahir* and *Batin* not only are a way to think about this balance, but also are intended to help individuals live in balance. Such teachings are integral to reminding humankind that they are not above Creation.

The Qur'an also frequently calls upon humans to pay attention to *ayat* or signs of the Creator's existence. *Ayat* refers to the actual verses of the Qur'an and the Creator's outward manifestations. In the *Encyclopedia of the Qur'an*, McAuliffe (2006) emphasizes that the Qur'an repeatedly insists that Creator is offering *ayat* that "manifest all we need to know" (p. 1). *Ayat* is understood as a way to summon Creation back to Truth. *Ayat* can manifest as signs of nature and the historical narration of the Creator to come into relationship with Creation (McAuliffe, 2006). A disconnect between meaning and form interferes with interpretation and undermines the notion that human beings have been bestowed with the responsibility of *Ashraf al-Makhluqat* to safeguard the life of all beings and ensure the collective survival of all. Rumi conceptualized ecological principles based on this ethic and explained that nature guides and instructs us to refrain from the compartmentalization that occurs when we intellectualize our being (Clarke, 2003).

Sacred Ecological Philosophies amongst Indigenous Wisdom Traditions

The wisdom that flows from Indigenous spiritualities teaches that all life forms are interconnected (Basso, 1996; Cardinal & Hildebrandt, 2000; B. Cardinal, 2014; Hanohano, 1999; LaBoucane-Benson et al., 2012; ; Northwest Territories, Education, Culture and Employment, 1993; Simpson, 2014). Living and non-living entities are brought into being through a Creator. It is understood that the Creator bestows all beings with unique gifts, knowledge systems, and rules of living to support balance and harmony. For these reasons, human beings are not the arbiters of life and living, but rather are beholden to other life forms. Peter Hanohano also explicates these sentiments regarding the importance of honouring Mother Earth as a living being. Hanohano (1999) draws upon McGaa (1990) to outline,

> Our survival is dependent on the realization that Mother Earth is a truly holy being, that all things in this world are holy and must not be violated, and that we must share and be generous with one another. You may call this thought by whatever fancy words you wish – psychology, theology, sociology, or philosophy – but you must think of Mother Earth as a living being. Think of your fellow men and women

as holy people who were put here by the Great Spirit. Think of being related to all things! With the philosophy in mind as we go on with our environmental ecology efforts, our search for spirituality, and our quest for peace, we will be far more successful when we truly understand the Indians' respect for Mother Earth. (pp. 208–209)

These insights indicate the ways in which connectivity is made possible through a Creator that unites all forms. This insight is integral to understand if we seek to come into deeper relationships with Indigenous worldviews and spiritualities. Forgetting the specific roles that all life forms play and their shared connection to spirit results in imbalance and disharmony.

The Wisdom-Guided Curricular and Pedagogical Context of Aboriginal Studies 30

I experienced much imbalance during my K–12 experiences because I was forced to invisibilize the ways in which Islam guides me in my daily living. Therefore, this work is guided by what was missing from my own education through the course's underpinnings in holistic sensibilities that centre the Spirit. The course creation process initially commenced with three individuals who were seeking to create a programme of studies. These individuals came alongside Elders, community members, teachers, and students from Dene, Cree, Saulteaux, and Blackfoot territories (E. Goodstriker, personal communication, May 2, 2017). This guidance was conceptualized as representing the threads of history, spirituality, cultures, and traditions. Particular threads had more information than others. Consequently, individuals from all nations across Alberta were consulted for guidance. Conversations across the province were particularly guided by wisdom keepers and teachers. These conversations and curricular formations were inspired by the insights that flowed from ceremony. Reconnecting with oneself and other life forms while partaking in ceremony guided how curriculum development was understood and what it was for.

For these reasons, the Aboriginal Studies Programme of Studies is guided by holism. Some of these philosophical commitments include:

1. Enables all students to demonstrate an understanding that societies are made up of individuals, but each individual has a responsibility to the well-being of the society.
2. Illustrates the importance of the spiritual nature of Aboriginal peoples and their relationship with all things in the universe.
3. Helps all students to develop respect for the environment and commitment to use resources wisely.
4. Helps all students to appreciate values related to their personal, ethical and spiritual beliefs.

(Alberta Education, 2002, p. 2)

These philosophical commitments convey how Aboriginal Studies is guided by the ethics of interconnectivity, kinship, and Spirit. These philosophies supported course activities which were grounded in traditional teachings and conceptions of treaty relationships.

Introducing Alissa, Rose, Levi, and Chauntelle

Former Aboriginal Studies 30 student research participants were invited to write characterizations of themselves during the research process. The intent of this was to ensure that students were represented on their own terms. A brief overview of each participant is provided next to understand who they are and how they were impacted by the course throughout the program.

Chauntelle Atcheynum is from Sweetgrass First Nation. She is pursuing a career in teaching the Cree language to youth and developing a language immersion program for educational institutions. She is passionate about the implementation of Indigenous worldviews into the education system as well as decolonization efforts within these institutions. For a long time, she distanced herself from her culture and its traditions. It took much courage for her to return to her roots and accept who she is. She has chosen to embrace and empower other individuals to honour and love who they are and where they come from. She seeks to advocate for Aboriginal communities and their healing process.

Alissa James is from Alberta. She was 19 years old at the time of the study. She wants to help students of various capabilities succeed and thrive in an educational curriculum that is otherwise stagnant and slowly developing. Alissa comes from a family of 11 with 8 other siblings. She had a very hectic childhood. While she often changed schools and homes, the one constant she shared was her culture. Her family has ties in both Dene and Plains Cree cultures, but the lifestyle she grew up with was very much Cree oriented.

Levi Matthews describes himself as having German, Irish, English, and Métis ancestry. He is significantly guided by Christian sensibilities in his life. Levi was studying political sciences at the time of the research.

Rose Salvador was born in the Philippines and migrated to Canada when she was 17. She is was an English major student at the time of the study. She sees herself as an individual who would prefer to follow than to lead others. She loves giving her true opinions when asked. She has a Filipino, Chinese, and Spanish background, which has made her more open to different ways of thinking.

The Research Process

This research inquiry is guided by an emerging form of métissage. Métissage is a theory and textual practice that beckons researchers and audiences "to create plural selves that thrive on ambiguity and multiplicity" (Chambers & Hasebe-Ludt, 2008, p. 3). The origin of métissage is the Latin word

Mixiticus, which means "the weaving of cloth from different fibers" (Hasebe-Ludt & Jordan, 2010, p. 3). Greek mythology describes Métis as the earliest form of wisdom and a trickster with transformative powers who resisted purity by weaving textiles. Following Donald's practices of métissage (2009), I conceptualize and enact métissage as a way to guide the shift from identity to more deepened enactments of relationality. I situate ethical relationality as a way of life through my connections with Islam and Cree philosophies. Islam is often described as "a way life." My growing connections with Cree sensibilities have guided my understanding of ethical relationality as a way of life. Reconnecting with the insights that flow from sacred ecological holistic insights remind me that I am connected with the Creator and Creation in all moments.

Research Design and Enactments

The spirit and intent of coming alongside four Aboriginal Studies 30 students was to learn from the underlying sensibilities that guided their interpretations of difference. In order to honour the métissage and hermeneutic philosophical underpinnings of this work, my research design intentionally focused on students' former engagement with specific facets of the course as shared commonalities and engagement with two new shared activities. The purpose of this was to circle back to former experiences in the course and to create anew in response to our new experiences.

Research activities and their accompanying questions were specifically created to reconnect with, address, and give voice to the holism that undergirds Aboriginal Studies 30. The intention of each question was to simultaneously address how we have been typically taught to address matters of relationality, connectivity, and difference, and juxtapose this with what was "lifted" through coming alongside holistic-guided curricular and pedagogical approaches in Aboriginal Studies 30. Activity 1 explored "how might the four directions as Elder Cardinal explained them inform our understanding of respectful relationships in the place of Edmonton" through the Elder's loving guidance. Following our activity session, the students and I came together for a research conversation and shared our experiences, insights gleaned, and overall connecting experiences. Activity 2 addressed "how do we understand (or come to terms with) who we are in the place of Edmonton." This exploration frontloaded students' learnings surrounding the histories and implications of the Indian Residential School System and engagements with the Truth and Reconciliation Commission's Calls to Action. The purpose of this question was to investigate how we understand and articulate who we are in connection to shared histories and memories (McLeod, 2007; Stanley, 2006). Activity 3 examined "in what ways does the land here teach us who we are in relation to each other" (Basso, 1996; Chambers, 2006; Simpson, 2014). The aim of this question was to come into deeper connections with kinship relational networks and what this teaches in our daily lives. What might we learn from not only drawing upon historical teachings of place, but also engaging with sacred ecological insights in embodied ways? The students and I participated in a River Valley walk led by Dr. Dwayne Donald in which sacred ecological teachings were shared in relationship to the places we visited as a group. The River Valley walk was followed by a conversation surrounding our experiences with the walk and insights regarding what sacred ecology teaches us about differences and sameness. Lastly, Activity 4 addressed the question "what does equality mean to you." This exploration was connected to how Aboriginal Studies 30 addresses differences between Indigenous and Canadian readings of equality. The intention of investigating this question as a shared research conversation was to open up the confluence of personal readings of equity, difference, and belonging in connection to Aboriginal Studies 30's representation of difference and its tensionalities within Canadian liberal multiculturalism.

Reconnecting with Life-Giving Energy: Alissa's, Rose's, Levi's, and Chauntelle's Experiences with Learning from Sacred Ecology

The following insights highlight the student participants' learnings regarding opportunities to learn from the generative energy of sacred ecology. As this section will express, reconnecting with life-giving energies brings forth a form of remembering and feelings of deep love and responsibility that critical personalistic and individualistic approaches overlook. Experiencing and connecting with the wisdom that flows from sacred notions of difference may teach us to believe in our spirit and to nurture and grow change.

The métissage that follows intends to reawaken that which has become dormant and is necessary to better connect with ourselves and our relations in deeper ways. Its textual representations and the truths that arise from it express a way of "doing" and understanding difference differently. The text conveys the curricular and pedagogical importance of holistic insights in guiding individual and collective enactments of healing, reconnecting with kinship, and trusting in embodied understandings as sources which can help to "lift us up" and renew our commitments in this shared life together. This embodied process entails attending to complexity as a way to open up the heart and mind (Cardinal, 2014; Rahman, 2013; Virani, 2002). There is much at stake if we continue to depend solely on intellectualized approaches to life and living, connectivity, and survival.

A curriculum dialogue is presented via métissage. The following section begins with two purposeful Rumi poetry selections. These pieces were chosen on the basis of guidance they offer specifically pertaining to connecting with embodied insights and living in ways that honour our shared sacred ecological roots. Learning from Rumi's poetry presents an opportunity to counter prevailing Islamophobic images of Muslims in the media (Akbari,

2016), the hidden curriculum of schools, and provincially mandated texts. Drawing upon Rumi's poetry to begin each section is also meant to facilitate a dialogue between Sufic and Cree wisdom sensibilities and their different sacred ecological insights. The intention here is to encourage creativity and restore deeper connectivity through learning from the traditions' convergent and divergent sacred ecological teachings. This approach shifts our understanding beyond normalized monolithic representations of who we are and reminds that we are gifted with individual and collective agency. Rumi's poetry is also drawn upon to invite readers to engage in interpretive acts themselves from the places that they are currently situated and partake in their own meaning-making alongside the insights of former Aboriginal Studies students. Following Rumi's poetry, excerpts from research conversations with four former Aboriginal Studies students are shared. These excerpts will be presented beginning with Alissa, followed by Rose, Levi, and, lastly, Chauntelle. An interpretation will proceed with each selection of text. The student interpretations that follow will arise from the shared questions . This is to honour the hermeneutical priority of the question that Gadamer (1975) emphasizes.

Following the sharing of the question, each interpretation will begin with dwelling in Rumi's poetry and unpacking his words in relation to Qur'anic holistic insights. Next, I will ponder the words of each participant and how their experiences with holism in Aboriginal Studies and insights gleaned from research activities informed their understandings of emerging themes. The holistic themes that manifested during this study include healing, balance, and kinship. I will also elucidate thematic unities between participants' experiences and shared insights with Rumi's poetry as a way to illuminate what the false universalism of liberalism misses on curricular and pedagogical landscapes. Lastly, a curriculum conversation will express the significance of student participants' insights in relationship to curriculum and pedagogy. This conversation will be shared at the end of each section of the métissage. The purpose of dwelling in participants' voices and revisiting their understandings throughout the braiding process is to honour the integrity of each participant and enact the organic and transformative ethics espoused by métissage.

One Task

There is one thing in the world that you must never forget. You may forget everything else except that one thing, without any cause for worry. However, if you remember and take care of everything else but forget that one thing, you will have accomplished nothing. It is as though a king were to send you to a village on a specific mission. You go and perform a hundred other tasks, but if you neglect to take care of the task for which you were sent, it is as though you did absolutely nothing. The human being has come into the world for a particular

purpose. If he does not accomplish that purpose, he will have done nothing at all. We offered the trust to the heavens, and the earth, and the mountains: and they refused to undertake it, and were afraid of it, but the human being undertook it – but, surely, he has been unjust to himself, and foolish (31:72).
[Fihi ma Fihi: Discourse 4]

(Jalaluddin Rumi, in Helminski and Helminski, 2012, *The Rumi Daybook*, p. 24)

The Truth Within Us

I was a fair orchard,
Full of trees and fruit
And vines and greenery. A Sufi there
sat with eyes closed, his head upon his knee,
Sunk deep in meditation mystical.
"Why," asked another, "do you not behold
These signs of God the Merciful displayed
Around you, which He bids us contemplate?"
"The signs," he answered, "I behold within,
Without is nothing but symbols of the Signs."
What is beauty in the world? The image,
Like quivering laughs reflected in a stream,
Of that eternal orchard which abides
Unwithered in the hearts of the Perfect Men.

(Jalaluddin Rumi, in Dunn et al., 2010, *The Illustrated Rumi*, p. 2)

I think difference does create more difference. But I think it's done in a way in order for people to find where they belong. The right to belong and feel accepted is a feeling sought after by all lifelong but is never far away.

I think that in some way we are connected. If we weren't we would be annihilated already. Like we wouldn't be here if we weren't connected by nature in some ways.

Water makes up everyone's body. And like people say the water that people bathed in the 1700s is the water that we could be drinking today. It just shows that everything is truly a cycle and is connected. I don't think that our differences are a hindrance to that at all. I think that we should celebrate the differences and similarities because everything is about balance in that regard.

We are not perfect beings. We are filled with error and faults and mistakes and that's how we learn, and if we were surrounded by a world that is perfect and looked identical and the same and every tree grew at the same place, what would we learn from? We would destroy ourselves. The land is different in every place.

How does kinship guide deepen understandings of connectivity?

As I revisit Rumi's breath-taking poem "One Task," I am reminded of Rose's generative insights regarding her experiences in Aboriginal Studies 30 as a bundle carrier. The Ontario Centre of Excellence for Child and Youth Mental Health (n.d.) explains that bundles play an integral role in the health and well-being of many Indigenous peoples. Physical bundles refer to a collection of sacred items, including eagle feathers and medicines, that are important to share with others. Bundles are often carried by Indigenous peoples attending ceremony. Particular Indigenous cultures hold the belief that

> when a child is born they come into the world with a spiritual bundle which holds all of the gifts the Creator gave to them. Both physical and spiritual bundles serve the purpose of helping a person to engage with creation in a healthy and balanced way.
>
> (The Ontario Centre for Excellence for Child and Youth Mental Health, n.d. para. 1)

Rose was gifted with a bundle from Jodi Stonehouse, who co-produces an Indigenous radio programme called *Acimowin* on CJSR Radio in Alberta. Rose shared (personal communication, November 2014):

> It is such an honor [to receive a bundle]. It is the greatest gift that an Aboriginal person can give. It is an experience that no one can take from you. You have it for life. I feel so proud that she picked me. I cried when Jodi gave it to me. I can't explain why it means so much to me. It makes me more compassionate. It's not just about me. It's a European perspective, a Spanish perspective, an Aboriginal perspective. I see it as all perspectives going together. When I experience like this it makes me more honest with myself. It is different from just reading about it.

Rose's compelling insights convinced me to reconsider the positioning of perspectival approaches to difference and the extent to which they can promote unity. My ability to engage with Rose's words at the time was rather limited because I was in the process of beginning to reconnect with myself and sacred ecological insights. I understand more clearly today that Rose also helped me to reawaken within myself what had become dormant in my memory and being. While certain K–12 experiences provided me with opportunities to learn from culturally responsive pedagogy, this curricular approach's birth from the civil rights movement, focus on supporting academic achievement and incorporating culture (Ladson-Billings, 1995a, 1995b, 2014) did not allow for me to reconnect with and learn from my own embodiment and that which gifts life. While culturally responsive practices attended to conceptions of self, social relations, and conceptions of knowledge (Ladson-Billings, 1995a), they were unable to deconstruct how colonialism has and continues to impact the education system (Pirbhai-Illich et al., 2017), or able to counter the universalization of one way to live within the purview of neoliberal curricular priorities. Although these practices are essential and well-intentioned, the axioms that undergird culturally relevant pedagogy are still primarily rooted in a capitalistic ethic that seeks entry into the labour market, and do not directly support healing from the ways in which colonialism denies the relationship from the mind, heart, and spirit, and from those who look different from us (Donald, 2010). Rose's insights amplify the urgency and possibility to attend to a curriculum of embodiment on curricular and pedagogical sites as a way to unlearn colonialism and recover relationship. Her words speak to the gift of the "one task" as a trustworthy teacher that can inspire openness to others and a deepened sense of connectivity and convey how holistic insights offer generative understandings of difference.

Rumi shares,

> There is one thing in the world that you must never forget. You may forget everything else except that one thing, without any cause for worry. However, if you remember and take care of everything else but forget that one thing, you will have accomplished nothing.

Drawing upon Rose's words and learning from Cree philosophies, I interpret Rumi's words as directly expounding the Qur'anic teaching of *Ashraf al-Makhluqat*. *Ashraf al-Makhluqat* is understood as a sacred gift from Allah that entrusts human beings with the lofty responsibility of ensuring that Creation remains protected, well taken care of, and most importantly that there is balance and harmony between all life forms. This responsibility is imbued in humility and meaning-making that can be espoused through learning from the *ayat* (signs) embedded in our relations. These signs inspire communication amongst our relations that renew life and actively promote and sustain connectivity. Shainool Jiwa (n.d.) expresses this thought and shares that "one of the key manifestations of God's *rahma* (mercy) is the communication with humanity. Divine communication occurs through the numerous *ayat* (signs) in creation and through the prophets" (para. 10). This *rahma* (mercy) through the appearance of difference as it arises from *ayat* (signs) is a deep source of guidance but also a task that requires careful attention. Jiwa further underscores that from Qur'anic sensibilities, human beings are gifted as the most Noble of Creation because they are appointed as Allah's *Khalifat* or vicegerents on earth. This designation positions human beings as the "care-taker[s] of Creation and [as] accountable for its well-being to their Creator, who is the sustainer of the worlds" (Jiwa, n.d., para. 9). Rumi subsequently refers to this Qur'anic cosmological teaching as the "one task" that ought not be forgotten. Thus, Rumi emboldens our human tendency to forget that our life and living is in fact beholden to other entities. He compels us to reflect upon the potential results of forgetting this one task.

Rumi's poem "The Truth Within Us" similarly evokes remembering the Divine granting of difference as gifted through *ayat* (signs). Rumi narrates this poem via an exchange between a Sufi and another individual. Trees and fruit sit before the Sufi who is sitting in deep meditation. An individual asks the Sufi, "Why do you not behold these signs of God the merciful displayed around you, which He bids us contemplate?" The Sufi answers that he carries these *ayat* within. I interpret this exchange as calling for the importance of inner interpretation, which is a key theme in Rumi's poetry and the *wahkohtowin* teaching emphasizing that what surrounds us is inside of us. Rumi is suggesting that meaning is lost when the different sources of guidance are merely treated as symbols.

Alissa's, Rose's, Levi's, and Chauntelle's experiences of deeper expressions and enactments of connectivity are informed by the holistic underpinnings of Aboriginal Studies 30 and partaking in a River Valley walk for this research study under the guidance of Dr. Dwayne Donald. Alissa attends to her initial presumptions that difference begets more difference but also is a deep source of belonging. Rose frontloads nature as a source of connection that ensures the continuity of life. Levi specifically addresses how water is often taken for granted as a sacred gift and teaches us about connectivity in the midst of difference. Chauntelle expresses how sacred ecological insights inform how she understands errors and faults as profound instructors on life and living.

Alissa initially states that "difference does create more difference." She however proceeds to share that the pervasiveness of difference is needed to help "people to find where they belong." Her words indicate that the integrity of all beings ought to be honoured as they work towards acceptance and belonging in their own ways. Of noteworthy attention in Alissa's ponderings is her emphasis that the work of belonging and acceptance is "lifelong." Matters of living and beingness cannot be resolved in fleeting moments. Perhaps the sacred ecological ethics she was enmeshed in through her Aboriginal Studies experiences and while partaking in the River Valley walks inspired this conception of time as integral to matters of belonging and connection.

Rose speaks to connection in another way through emphasizing that without nature we might very likely be annihilated already. She shares, "We wouldn't be here if we weren't connected to nature in some ways." Her insights open up Rumi's emphasis on paying attention to the one task. Her words also emphasize that connecting with our kinship relational networks in the places we reside teaches us what we need to live well (Donald, 2016). Rose's words speak to a holistic understanding of connectivity that makes evident the pedagogical nature of sacred ecological philosophies.

Levi also draws upon holistic-guided sacred ecological insights which inform his interpretations of connectivity. He reflects on the teaching that all bodies are made of water, and people bathe in water and also drink water. His learnings from the sacred gift of water help him to articulate an understanding of connectivity that holds our relations together. Levi's understandings of "water" as a gift can be understood as an *ayat* or sign regarding that which connects us all and ensures the continuity of life. Levi further explains that the different ways in which water supports life and living conveys the understandings that "everything is truly a life cycle." Drawing upon inspiration from these holistic-guided sacred ecological insights, Levi understands the simultaneous presence of similarities and differences as another opportunity to instil balance. His words indicate a contemplation of *ayat* in an inner sense which Rumi continuously advocates for. It is Levi's kinship with other life-giving entities that invites inner reflection and a deepened sense of connectivity.

Chauntelle's conceptions of connectivity and generativity are inspired by holistic-guided sacred ecological insights. She shares the dangers that would arise "if we were surrounded by a world that is perfect and looked identical and the same." Chauntelle ponders, if "every tree grew at the same place what would we learn from them?" She indicates that the presence of sameness would inevitably lead to the destruction of ourselves. Chauntelle's words also display thematic unity with Rumi's poetry because she is deeply dwelling in the *ayat* (signs) of meaning-making that grant life. Her dwelling in these insights and alongside her kinship relational network reminds her that "the land is different in every place" and that there is a deeper reason for this. Chauntelle's holistic readings of connectivity also reposition and help us to explore the differences that arise through error and faults, which have transformative potential that supports openness.

Alissa's, Rose's, Levi's, and Chauntelle's perceptions uphold the importance of inner dwelling as a source of guidance and meaning-making in their lives. Inner dwelling, according to their experiences, is inspired by connecting with kinship or relational networks that honour connections to our more-than-human relatives. Their insights share thematic unity with Rumi's emphasis of upholding the one task and holding signs within oneself to generate deeper meaning that reduces the separation between all life forms.

Forward Together: Curricular and Pedagogical Implications

The promotion of a particular form of survival that is promised through "becoming somebody" and acquiring "material recognition" can lead to imbalance that is difficult to recover from. The student participants' experiences indicate that a loss of self is perpetuated by forgetting our enmeshment with our kinship relational networks and subsequently the one task that Rumi opens up. This loss of self and our relations also promotes the concealment of deeper meaning that can guide individual and collective transformation as evidenced by the student participants' experiences of healing. Enhancing the "curriculum as planned" (Aoki, 1991, p. 39) or strictly adhering to mandated curricular outcomes, through adherence to epistemological notions of difference that are assimilated by anthropocentric conceptions of sameness and unity, interferes with the potential for students to connect with their embodied knowledges. This distance from kinship and embodied knowledge ensures that learnings that are meant to promote greater openness to others remain dormant in life and living. The student participants' experiences reveal that holism enlivens memory and brings to life what is disseminated in curricular and pedagogical contexts in ways that the "curriculum as planned" (Aoki, 1991) cannot. Their connections to holistic-guided sacred ecological insights invited a recovery of memory that offered guidance on how to become better human beings. This is why Aboriginal Studies 30 was life-changing for Alissa, Rose, Levi, and Chauntelle. The knowledge they acquired from reconnecting with themselves through holistic insights was life-changing because it became a part of their embodiment. The student participants were not isolated from their learnings but rather became enmeshed in difference with their whole bodies. Alissa, Rose, Levi, and Chauntelle remembered their enmeshment, which resulted in a return to inner dwelling and the cultivation of an awareness that was transformative and life-giving. Remembering that we are not "isolated creatures with isolated thoughts" (Morris, 2002, p. 581) through reconnecting with our shared ecological roots, as guided by holism, offers ways in which balance can be restored on curricular and pedagogical contexts. Survival ought not be limited to the confines of individualism and materialism but can also be understood and enacted in ways that promote recovery from our shared ecological amnesia and safeguards all of our relations.

These foundational insights have much to offer to the future of curriculum and pedagogy. Firstly, reinterpreting my subjective experiences of holism in relation to Cree philosophies brings forth a manifestation of holism that does not erase Spirit in fears of secular institutional impositions. Secondly, this work recovers how Islam is also a holistic tradition that can inspire living wisely and well by dwelling in Rumi's poetry. Thirdly, this work proposes a métissage through dialogue between Cree and Sufic sensibilities that tries to aesthetically represent what is left out on pedagogical sites when holism is abandoned. Lastly, this work invites readers to take seriously the curricular and pedagogical significance of healing and how holistic insights in this regard can promote wellness and relationships that inspire us to acknowledge and seek guidance from the transformative beauty of our relations that are always here and beckon us to live in accordance with the "one task."

References

Alberta Education. (2002). *Aboriginal studies 10-20-30*. Retrieved from http://education.alberta.ca/media/654004/abor102030.pdf

Akbari, E. (2016). Rumi: A cosmopolitan counter-narrative to Islamophobia. *Journal of Cultural Research in Art Education, 33*, 48–67.

Aoki, T. (1991). Teaching as indwelling between two curriculum worlds. In T. Aoki (Ed.), *Inspiriting curriculum and pedagogy: Talks to teachers* (pp. 7–10). Department of Secondary Education, University of Alberta.

Asch, M. (2014). *On being here to stay: Treaties and aboriginal rights in Canada.* University of Toronto Press.

Basso, K. (1996). *Wisdom sits in places: Landscapes and language among the Western Apache.* University of New Mexico Press.

Cardinal, B. (2014). *Conversations and teachings in EDSE 601.* Enoch Cree Nation.

Cardinal, H., & Hildebrandt, W. (2000). *Treaty elders of Saskatchewan: Our dream is that our peoples will one day be clearly recognized as nations.* University of Calgary Press.

Chambers, C. (2006). "Where do I belong?" Canadian curriculum as passport home. *Journal of the American Association for the Advancement of Curriculum Studies, 2,* 1–21.

Chambers, C., & Hasebe-Ludt, E. (with Donald, D., Hurren, W., Leggo, C., & Oberg, A.). (2008). *Métissage*: A research praxis. In J. G. Knowles & A. Cole (Eds.), *Handbook of the arts in qualitative research: Perspectives, methodologies, examples, and issues* (pp. 141–153). Sage.

Clarke, L. (2003). The universe is alive: Nature in the Masnavi of Jalal al-Din Rumi. In R. C. Foltz, F. M. Denny, & A. Baharuddin (Eds.), *Islam and ecology: A bestowed trust.* Harvard University Press.

Consciousness. (2021). In *Online etymology dictionary.* Retrieved from https://www.etymonline.com/search?q=consciousness

Dei, G. J. S. (1996). *Anti-racism education : Theory and practice.* Fernwood Pub.

Donald, D. (2009). *The pedagogy of the Fort: Curriculum, aboriginal-Canadian relations and indigenous métissage* [Unpublished doctoral dissertation]. University of Alberta.

Donald, D. (2010). On what terms can we speak? Retrieved from http://vimeo.com/15264558

Donald, D. (2016). From what does ethical relationality flow? An *Indian* act in three artifacts. In J. Seidel & D. Jardine (Eds.), *The ecological heart of teaching: Radical tales of refuge and renewal for classrooms and community* (pp. 10–16). Peter Lang Publishing.

Donald, D. (2019). Homo economicus and forgetful curriculum: Remembering other ways to be a human being. In H. T. Tomlins-Janke, S. Styre, S. Lilley, & D. Zinga (Eds.), *Indigenous education: New direction in theory and practice* (pp. 103–119). University of Alberta Press.

Dunn, P., Dunn Mascetti, M., & Nicholson, R. A. (2010). *The illustrated Rumi: A treasury of wisdom from the poet of the soul.* HarperCollins.

Ellsworth, E. (1989). Why doesn't this feel empowering? Working through the repressive myths of critical pedagogy. *Harvard Educational Review, 59*(3), 297–325.

Gadamer, H.-G. (1975). *Truth and method.* Seabury Press. (Original work published 1960)

Hanohano, P. (1999). Native epistemology: Restoring harmony and balance in education. *Canadian Journal of Native Education, 23*(2), 206–219.

Hasebe-Ludt, E., & Jordan, N. (Eds.). (2010). May we get us a heart of wisdom: Life writing across knowledge traditions. *Transnational Curriculum Inquiry, 7*(2), 1–4.

Helminski, K., & Helminski, C. (2012). *The Rumi daybook: 365 Poems and teachings from the beloved Sufi master*. Shambhala.

Islamic Sciences and Research Academy Australia. (2012). Environmental ethics in Islam. Retrieved from http://www.ceosyd.catholic.edu.au/Parents/Religion/RE/ Documents/Environmental%20Ethics%20in%20Islam%20P

Jiwa, S. (n.d.). Approaches to the Qur'an. Retrieved from https://iis.ac.uk/approaches -qur

Kasamali, Z. N. (2019). *Reconsidering difference: The curricular and pedagogical significance of holism*. [Doctoral Dissertation, University of Alberta]. https://era .library.ualberta.ca/items/5b50eb0d-6955-44b7-a68f-0bb88bd7f774

Kasamali, Z. (2020). Reconsidering difference: The curricular and pedagogical significance of holistic insights in the face of colonial exclusions. *Cultural and Pedagogical Inquiry*, 12(1), 216–228.

Kasamali, Z. (2021). Encountering difficult knowledge and the curricular and pedagogical significance of holism: Disrupting 9/11 orthodox accounts in social studies classrooms. *Annals of Social Studies Education Research for Teachers*, 2(1), 58–66.

Kasamali, Z. (2021). Throwing salt on wounds: Covid-19 and a curriculum of embodiment. *Prospects*, 51, 103–116.. https://doi.org/10.1007/s11125-021 -09561-x

Kumashiro, K. K. (2004). *Against common sense: Teaching and learning toward social justice*. Routledge Falmer.

LaBoucane-Benson, P., Gibson, G., Benson, A., & Miller, G. (2012). Are we seeking Pimatisiwin or creating Pomewin? Implications for water policy. *International Indigenous Policy Journal*, 3(3), 1–22.

Ladson-Billings, G. (1995a). Toward a theory of culturally relevant pedagogy. *American Educational Research Journal*, 32(3), 465–491.

Ladson-Billings, G. (1995b). But that's just good teaching! The case for culturally relevant pedagogy. *Theory into Practice*, 34(3), 159–165.

Ladson-Billings, G. (2014). Culturally relevant pedagogy 2.0: Aka the remix. *Harvard Educational Review*, 84(1), 74–84.

McAuliffe, J. D. (Gen. ed.). (2006). *Encyclopedia of the Qur'an*. Brill.

McGaa, E. (1990). *Mother earth spirituality: Native American paths to healing ourselves and our world*. HarperCollins.

McLeod, N. (2007). *Cree narrative memory: From treaties to contemporary times*. Purich Pub.

Morris, M. (2002). Ecological consciousness and curriculum. *Journal of Curriculum Studies*, 34(5), 571–587.

Northwest Territories. (1993). *Dene Kede: Education, a Dene perspective*. Department of Education, Culture and Employment, Government of the Northwest Territories.

Paine, R. (1999). Aboriginality, multiculturalism and liberal rights philosophy. *Ethnos*, 64(3), 325–350.

Pirbhai-Illich, F., Pete, S., & Martin, F. (2017). Culturally responsive pedagogies: Decolonization, indigeneity and interculturalism. In F. Pirbhai-Illich, S. Pete, & F. Martin (Eds.), *Culturally responsive pedagogy: Workings towards decolonization, indigeneity and interculturalism* (pp. 3–25). Palgrave Macmillan.

Rahman, I. J. (2013). Spiritual gems of Islam: Insights and practices from the Qur'an Hadith, Rumi and Muslim teaching stories to enlighten the heart and mind. SkyLight.

Simpson, L. (2014). Land as pedagogy: Nishnaabe intelligence and rebellious transformation. Decolonization: Indigeneity, *Education and Society*, 3(3), 1–25.

Smith, D. G. (2006). Trying to teach in a season of great untruth: Globalization, empire and the crises of pedagogy. Sense.

Smith, D. G. (2014). *Teaching as a practice of wisdom*. Bloomsbury Academic.

Some, M. (1994). *Of water and spirit: Ritual, magic, and initiation in the life of an African Shaman*. Tarcher/Putnam.

Stanley, T. (2006). Whose public? Whose memory? Racisms, grand narratives and Canadian history. In R. Sandwell (Ed.), *To the past: History education, public memory, and citizenship in Canada* (pp. 32–49). University of Toronto Press.

The Ontario Centre for Excellence for Child and Youth Mental Health. (n.d.). Bundles. Retrieved from https://www.cymh.ca/en/index.aspx

Turner, D. A. (2006). *This is not a peace pipe: Towards a critical indigenous philosophy*. University of Toronto Press.

Venn, C. (2002). Altered states: Post enlightenment cosmopolitanism and transmodern socialities. *Theory, Culture, and Society*, 19(1–2), 65–80.

Virani, N. (2002). " I am the Nightingale of the Merciful": Rumi's Use of the Qur'an and Hadith. *Comparative Studies of South Asia, Africa and the Middle East*, 22(1), 100–111.

Zinnbauer, B. J., Paragament, K. I., Cole, B., Rye, M. S., Butter, E. M., Belavich, T. G., Hipp, K. M., Scott, A. B., & Kadar, J. L. (1997). Religion and spirituality: Unfuzzying the fuzzy. *Journal for the Scientific Study of Religion*, 36(4), 549–564.

11 Easing Anxiety for Adults in Higher Education

Regaining Self within Subversive, Interdisciplinary Bibliotherapy, and Visual Journaling

Christina Belcher

As a professor in education, during my 2020 classes I recognized a change not only in student anxiety levels, but in the normativity of what defines anxiety in the minds of those experiencing it. For example, as a child, living within a modernist worldview, I understood anxiety to occur when I was concerned about a particular thing or event in context. My parents taught me to resolve anxiety by face-to-face discourse with parents, peers, or wiser, experienced acquaintances, so that I could find a path forward. Anxiety was viewed as a normative part of life.

Since the onset of COVID-19, the view of anxiety has moved from being a normative part of life to being a victimizing condition. A change in normativity occurs when anxiety moves from being a part of life as one deals with a concerning event to that of a psychological condition.

The American Psychological Association (2021) explains anxiety and stress as cooperatives. Though both are emotional responses, stress erupts after something triggers anxiety. Pain and suffering can ensue if stressors are not acknowledged or mediated. My students did not appear to have scaffolding to assist them in understanding that anxiety did not have to remain permanent.

In addition to stress and anxiety, a third component, culture, has now embraced a transhumanist worldview. Although I began this study unaware of why that would matter, it became more apparent as this study progressed, appearing as an epistemological shudder (Charteris, 2014); an aha moment caught by surprise in our narrative journey. As a professor, I felt responsible for assisting these students in overcoming a state of anxiety that would hinder their learning, view of self, belonging within a sense of place, and identity.

My professorial role in this process was essential. My goals involved forgetting past andragogy, implementing visual journals (VJs) in higher education, considering the bibliotherapeutic benefits of deep reading in literature, pondering with students the role of being human in culture, and a goal of reducing pain and suffering during the new horizon of a pandemic. This

DOI: 10.4324/9781003205296-14

involved changing some of the longstanding narratives of what schooling was for while implementing new ones.

A mutually dialogic, narrative journey within a learning community ensued. Literature will be interspersed as interactions unfold. Student interactions enfold the focal points of the chapter.

Context

This narrative takes place across a 13-week online semester course via the Google platform. Fourteen first-year education students will engage with literacy through poetry, fairy tales, picture books, and a selection of eight children's novels on themes of fantasy, contemporary fantasy, postmodern story, graphic novels, author study, science fiction, dystopian novels, special needs, and historical fiction. The work in class is crafted to reawaken the child in each reader through reflective reading, small and whole group discussions and interactions, assignment options, guiding questions about human *beings* and humans *doing*, and the art of visual journaling. These interactions provide a fertile generative landscape for learning about self-identity and life.

The Power of Words, Andragogy, and Story

Relationships between literacy, language, and power within social relationships and teaching/learning practices undergird research in critical literacy. However, I do not engage with the narrative of being critical as much as embracing narratives to form counternarratives to sociopolitical or institutional myths. Engaging critical literacy from the intention of liberating the voice and identity of the student for life inside and outside of the classroom through VJs, is not frequently used in higher education. I engage students to creatively stimulate meaningful dialogic discussion involving a thoughtful, reflective, and responsive interaction between literary text and life acts.

Discarding old andragogy and creating new procedures in assignments generated increased student voice and agency essential to creating a community of compassionate support where all voices become respected.

I began by altering my syllabus, making it a counternarrative to my former very detailed 12-page syllabus which included many institutional insertions. Although students did receive this larger syllabus the first class of online night class as required, class interactions demonstrated to me that it would not be helpful in a pandemic. Hence, I implemented a VJ format, with one page provided for each week of the course.

The course was revised to include options of choice for assignments so that students could have agency and power for submitted work. For example, students could choose between submitting a reflective essay on a novel or picture book, or a movie/book/article comparison, or writing a children's picture book for the format of a larger project. Reflections would involve

VJs and not solely essay. A quote from N. T. Wright (1996), rose to my mind:

> In our modern culture, we sometimes imagine that stories are kids' stuff – little illustrations – while abstract ideas are the real thing ... Stories are far more powerful than that. Stories create worlds. Tell the story differently and you change the world ... *stories were a way of getting to grips with reality.*

> (p. 36; emphasis added)

The reality I had to come to grips with in this course was a new one due to COVID-19. This bold statement by Wright was counternarrative to accepting that university education was only part of a knowledge economy, where knowledge was seen as information leading to vocational employment and efficiency. Intentionally, I steered my teaching goals and andragogy around why goals and questions on being human. My central themes became vulnerability and modelling, reflective practice, self-knowledge, and dialogue to reduce pain and suffering.

The Journey Begins

I initiated the first three-hour evening class session with two situating, introductory questions. Of 14 students in the class, in response to the first question "What should we know about you?" 5 stated: "I have [or am suffering from] high anxiety." In response to my second question, "What hinders you from learning?" one student in the online class responded:

> The syllabus! If I hear a prof say, "it is in the syllabus," I just feel I do not have time to read this and manage all this extra online time that online learning demands. I feel that I am not being heard as someone who may have a question for which the syllabus needs extension.

I perceived this comment as a stress trigger. That increased my student-declared anxiety level to six students: 42.8% of the class. Students were not saying they were "anxious" about an event that would pass; their "being" was being labelled as anxiety. In recognizing this, I set out to counter stress triggers by providing students with a sense of voice, self-identity, and small-group and whole-class conversations. My instructional design involved three guiding questions woven with themes of teacher modelling and guidance, visual journaling, dialogic discourse, and bibliotherapy.

Pain and Suffering: A Landscape for Engaging Questions

Question 1. How can my andragogy reduce anxiety by changing my approach to teaching and learning in an online format?

In addressing this question, I introduced students to VJs which can be found in Appendix A. I included an example of a VJ, which can be found in Appendix A, Box 11.1.

To reduce student anxiety, I instigated a dialogic interaction between visual journals with university literacy courses in *reading as a life act* (Belcher & Loerts, 2020; Blummer, 2015; Boche, 2014; Loerts & Belcher, 2019; Rowsell et al., 2012; Walsh, 2010). I define a *life act* as a response to the precept that we become the stories we tell; that all of life is made of stories we read, model, see, aspire to live, and present to others.

Question 2. How can the use of narrative sharing empower and strengthen students to overcome their fears by seeing anxiety from a distance through the course?

Authentic teaching, learning, and identity are evident in the work of Parker Palmer (1998, 2000, 2003, 2004; Palmer & Zajonc, 2010). Palmer believes that the identity of the teacher must be authentic, that teaching is more than technique, and that students must feel a sense of place and trust in the classroom. This requires ongoing, open-ended dialogic conversation. Lectures, when needed, must incorporate authentic voice and student engagement flowing from an awareness of student needs and agency.

Regie Routman (2018) declares that feeling confident in personal voice for students requires an excellence in providing meaningful questions and deep, reflective thinking about literature. She initiates this through story and personal experiences across the daily activities of teaching and learning to touch heads, hearts, and minds. This assists students in knowing who they are as people. Books become harbingers of hope.

In support of Routman (2018), in Baraister (2014) I read "all sorrows can be borne if you put them in a story or tell a story about them" (p. 45). McCulliss (2012) notes that bibliotherapy is derived from a combination of two Greek words: *biblion* (meaning "book") and *therapeia* (meaning "healing"). McCulliss and Chamberlain (2013, p. 13) state:

> Developmental bibliotherapy for children and youth has been defined as the use of literature to facilitate healthy social and emotional growth or maintain normal mental health. Developmental bibliotherapy is provided by educators who work with children and young adults. Miller (2009) further described bibliotherapy as "the process of using books to help youth and adolescents think about, understand, and work through social and emotional issues".
>
> (p. 260)

Literacy and anxiety are not separated within bibliotherapy (Carlson, 2001; Cornett & Cornett, 1980; Forgan, 2002; Jack & Ronan, 2008; Maich et al., 2016). This is a good posture for my goals.

Question 3. How can I assist students in becoming more confident in student voice and identity, so they can thrive?

Engaging the ethnographic work of Dorothy Smith (2005, 2006) on voice in educational settings revealed the inadequacy of sociological approaches in jumping to broad statements about the way the world operates. Doing so extinguishes or de-emphasizes the *particular* experiences of individuals and social groups, identified within *particular* institutional settings (Smith, 2005, pp. 27–33). Smith identified "problematics" in institutional life as ways of exploring deeper meaning: "[Traditional sociology] interprets the everyday and local events in terms of a framework originating in sociological and political discourse. Its conceptual structure displaces people, displaces their activities, displaces the social relations and organisation of their doings" (2005, p. 31). I gleaned from Smith that to reduce pain and suffering, a framework of safe, trusted, and honest dialogic conversation that engenders a feeling of belonging is required.

From Theory to Practice: Developing Authentic Voice to Combat Pain and Suffering

My first three online classes examined the genres of poetry, picture books, and fairy tales. These genres provided a safe sense of place for readers of any age to go back and remember things they loved about literacy and reading. This set the stage for deeper work, discussion, and presentations to follow. All members could see each other on the online platform.

Sometimes the start to class experienced a shared activity. For example, in our first class each student brought a piece of favourite childhood poetry and recited or read their favourite lines, expressing why these words were meaningful to them. At other times a question became the basis for the sharing VJs to extend discussion on a key concept. In this way everyone came prepared in advance of class to have a voice.

Each online night class began with a student reflection linking learning to life from the literary genre to be read on that evening. Ideas for deeper thinking were consistently included in the weekly VJs prior to class, so pre-thinking time was built into the response. Finally, a portion of the evening was allotted for class home groups of three or four students to have discussion on the novel or genre of the night in literature circles, and engage the heuristic by Charteris (2014) of "epistemological shudders" to report back on aha and oh no moments from the literature read. Following student feedback, I used open-ended questions to probe pertinent information they may have overlooked in a whole-group summary chat, rather than a lecture format.

Examples of Literary Engagement and Response

In student feedback, my guiding questions became interactive with the various conversations of the evening, the individual genres studied in class, and the stories examined in literature circles. Two questions of the day were helpful within the first four weeks of the course: *What are you learning and how does it make you feel?* And *What is the value of a story?* (Tables 11.1 and 11.2)

Responses revealed aspects of support for the VJs and for community building. Students became comfortable in engaging with me and each other. Being authentic and teaching with care and depth was something that students gravitated towards. The students frequently used VJs to process their reflective thoughts in novel studies after the midpoint of the course. These comments confirmed to me that story is bibliotherapeutic; never remaining at skin level with the reader.

I also noticed that student verbalizations were frequently in second person, addressing a community of learners, but with the addition of a

Table 11.1 What Are You Learning and How Does It Make You Feel?

Student Responses

- I am learning what it means to experience togetherness as a class, and not just as people in desks and chairs!

- I am learning that a teacher can be authentic to who she is and we can be authentic to who we are in a course.

- I am learning that I did not think I would like VJs because I am not good in art. Then I learned we were not evaluated on our art, but on our thinking process in making the art. Now I enjoy them.

- I am learning that thinking surfacely [word used by student] gives you information. Thinking deeply gives you wisdom.

- I am learning that how you [the professor] teach a class makes a difference in how meaningful it is to us.

- I think VJs are very therapeutic. I find doing something with my hands and mind to be very relaxing.

Table 11.2 What Is the Value of a Story?

Student Responses

- We can separate ourselves from the story, but also see ourselves in it in some way.
- Stories give us insight into someone else's head.
- Stories can bring clarity to how you feel and why.
- Stories provide caution towards the unknown.
- Stories do not feel like work to me. They feel like life through someone else's eyes.

- Stories help us decide what is true and realistic and what is not.
- Stories stay in your mind and are ongoing – you experience them as a recipient.
- Stories provide different perspectives on a problem.
- I think stories give us hope.
- I think stories bring out the philosophical side of me; the moral and ethical sides too.

personal perspective. Stories produce aesthetic, emotional responses, enabling the student to be in touch with self and others. I was seeing intentional pondering develop via story and narrative voices in conversation and reflection.

Engaging Novels

Our first novel, *Holes* (Sachar, 1998), provoked the question: *How do you cope with stress?* Students openly responded, stating that making lists, exercising, talking to family, music, reading, cleaning, and being outside helped in this area. I found it interesting that reading was on this list! When I asked why, a student replied: "Reading takes me out of who I am and shows me that at other times things were more difficult for people than they are now. They can be sort of a reality check!" These early connections demonstrated the significance of the question of the evening to open doors into voice for class members.

In one instance, anxiety was incognito, hiding in the question: "Doctor B., what do you do when you are stressed?" This noted the connection between stress and anxiety, showing that one was connected to the other in the thinking of the students. My response was I pray, and I try to do something kind for somebody else. One student said, "Oh, so if you pray, you sort of keep stress between yourself and God, and if you act, you do something to replace it that is beneficial." The class went on discussing stress, and concluded it is an inescapable part of life, and how you handle it makes a difference.

Student comments gave insight to the person that reads. These statements informed me that students can engage with story and feeling in ways in which they self-identify with what they read, hear, speak and share. The novel *Restart* (Korman, 2017) exposed this well.

Restart is about a boy with a severe head trauma after a concussion, and how he gradually remembers who he was and that defines who he becomes. He becomes a kinder human being, rather than the bully he was in his former days. One student in the class had a similar concussion following a car accident. He states in his VJ:

> I found this hard to read. It was like reliving everything and made me uncomfortable until I realized that it also gave opportunity for the insight to develop other ways of thinking about myself, so that I could become more than the label of my decreased memory; someone with a brain injury.

The student acquired more confidence in what he could achieve and focused less on what he could not during the course. This change in his confidence in class exposed that how I engage and provide questions provokes self-analysis and reduces anxiety in some way. It had done so for this young man.

The Invention of Hugo Cabret (Selznick, 2008) required a reflective reading and optional response between the article "I Have Forgotten How to Read" (Harris, 2018) in *The Globe and Mail*, or critiquing the difference between the book and its movie version (Table 11.3).

This option assignment really surprised me, as I thought digital natives would prefer the movie. They did not. Most preferred to discuss the article, suggesting that deeper thinking was more palatable to them than viewing, or that viewing, in essence, did not link to deeper thinking. The article reflection facilitated them in knowing more about themselves than the movie did.

Novels in this course crossed sociocultural lenses and beliefs over time (Table 11.4).

Table 11.3 Agency in Assignment Choice

The Invention of Hugo Cabret and Harris Article	*The Invention of Hugo Cabret* and Movie Comparison
• I noted that it is the distractions of online learning and media in general that cause me not to attend (pop up ads, side bars) as well as the speed of scrolling rather than needing to read a horizontal hard copy page.	• The biggest insight to me was that the conflict in the book is internal. The conflict in the movie is external. One is about the soul, the other about the action.
• This article has opened my eyes to recognize actual changes in my abilities to retain information and focus on something for more than a few minutes. What I found to be a refreshing sense of hope in this topic is when the writer says "So maybe that change into a cynical writer can be forestalled – if I can first correct my reading diet, remember how to read the way I once did. Not scan, not share, not excerpt – but read. Patiently, slowly, uselessly." I can change my reading diet.	• The characters in the movie are much older than those in the book, and the relationships in the movie are less authentic and more shallow. The deep friendship element is removed and substituted with weak romance.
• In my experience, having tangible pages to turn and touch improves my reading comprehension, reading speed, and I retain what I have read better.	• The book had a purpose and a beautiful way of exposing unprinted thought in the pictures. It was creative. The movie just did not have the same impact on me as reading the hard copy.
• Michael Harris hits the nail on the head when he says "To read was to shutter myself and, in so doing, discover a larger experience. I do think old, book-oriented styles of reading opened the world to me – by closing it. And new, screen-oriented styles of reading seem to have the opposite effect: They close the world to me, by opening it."	

Table 11.4 Worldview Lenses in Sociocultural Life

Cultural Lens	Definition
Modernism (following the Second World War till about the late 1970s)	Society's view of life gave value to the family, daily living, religion and norms of morality and justice. Society's lens respected parents, authority, and stressed being good to your neighbour.
Postmodernism (emerging in the 1980s till about 2000)	Postmodernism ushered in a form of critique and doubt. Criticize all and believe little. Society refuted past authority and history, believing in progressivism and individuality.
Post-postmodernism (2000–2018 or so as a cultural lens)	Society placed its hope in science and technology. Society's focus was often on what was wrong within society, not what was right. It valued rebellion and individual protest. It was angrier than the pessimistic doubt of the earlier postmodern social view.
Transhumanism (early political emergence in 2018; greatly enhanced by the COVID-19 pandemic)	Transhumanism ushered in the belief that being human was not enough. One must be digitally adapted and efficient in technology to have merit.

This awareness of social lenses emerged from a sociocultural discussion on the philosophy behind technology, reading excerpts out of Postman's book *Technopoly* (1993) and relating that to the connection of language in his other work *Conscientious Objections* (1988). This applied a *past, present, future lens*, identifying connections between language and technology, and technology and living life. The class really engaged in this, which was an unplanned but teachable event. Requesting further reading on the topic resulted in recommending *The End of Education* (Postman, 1995).

The class concluded that teachers should have a purpose and a plan for the use of technology in the classroom based on their own educational boundaries and reasons for use. In their responses, students were taking a moral stance in some of their arguments for and against technology which was a counternarrative on seeing technological use as an act of inattentiveness or entertainment, rather than a mindful use to engage learning. Students recognized this in their own ability to attend, to pay attention, while in online class. This discussion segued into how students would view their own andragogy for learning with technology, in an age promoting transhumanism.

Transhumanism is a philosophical concept very apt to COVID-19, that being human is not enough; one must be enhanced by technology (Gay, 2018). However, the technology has further implications on social life (Carr, 2010; Harris, 2014; Turkle, 2016; Twenge, 2017). Some of these implications are noted in my conclusions, but due consideration would require another chapter!

The postmodern novel *The Giver* (Lowry, 1993) included the question, *What do you appreciate most, or what troubles you about a dystopian novel?* This novel added consideration of beliefs regarding ethical situations (Table 11.5).

I noticed that there was eager participation and deeper interactive discourse and thinking going on about life and decision-making. Students were able to transport their thoughts to the issues raised and think deeply about what they, as humans, valued. The final novel was *The Book Thief* (Zusak, 2005). The question for the night was, *What does it mean to be fully human in a time of war?* (Table 11.6) Although this book rated in the top three for the course when students ranked the books from most to least valuable for teaching, little was said about it. One student said in a VJ:

> Our generation, and that of our parents have not as a country of citizens experienced war on this magnitude. It is a topic of sadness and yet of hope that we never have to see war again. After our grandparents die, there will be no one for this generation to remember as being involved in a war of this magnitude. We do not really know what to say but hope desperately that we never have to experience this in our country. What we liked most about this book, was the reality of character portrayal, and what we learned about life and death.

Table 11.5 What Do You Appreciate Most, or What Troubles You about a Dystopian Novel?

Appreciation	*Causes for Concern*
• Much like the genre of fairy tales, this effectively raised the binary opposites of good and evil for me.	• I found the coldness regarding topics of euthanasia and infanticide troubling, and a harbinger of what is occurring in the world today.
• I appreciated the aspect of memory and remembering as an enabler for good decision-making.	• I was saddened by the callousness of death, and by the impact of bad choices on others.
• I appreciated the importance of being unique, and making decisions for your life.	• It made me aware of the power of transferred knowledge, and how people may be remembered. I wonder if thinking in a past, present and future way would be a good way to live life, rather than acting and then regretting.
• I appreciated the aspect of passing things on to the next generation; like rites of passage perhaps.	
• I recognized the importance of citizenship, and what kind of citizen someone could become.	• The reality is that people can choose to be good or evil, and that reality is a consequence of personal choices.
• I was again aware of the fact that truth can be revealed in history through actions and consequences.	

Table 11.6 What Does It Mean to be Fully Human in a Time of War?

Student Responses	
• To be human, you must be authentic to who you are, despite circumstances. • Being human means, you have the strength to endure grief and stress in life. • I am saddened by human inhumanity to humans. And that is a good thing. I am also aware of the power of kindness to others as an act of grace.	• Being human means having compassion and being aware of others around you. • Being human means, we have the capacity to choose good over evil, which shows wisdom over unmindful reaction. • In this book, the narrator is Death. He says at the end, I am haunted by humans. He explains "I'm always finding humans at their best and worst. I see their ugly and their beauty, and I wonder how the same thing can be both" (p. 550). To me, it shows humans have the power of love in the face of death.

On our final night of class, we discussed the course, its accolades, and challenges. I asked the students if they felt as stressed at the end of the course as they did at the beginning. They said they did not. They attributed this change to a supportive, interactive learning community of their peers, time to give voice to what mattered to them, and a choice and variation in assignments.

Students verbally, or by note in summation of the course, recognized interpersonal, relational care and focus on student well-being as greatly impacting them. These comments assisted me in self-evaluation on my andragogy regarding putting the student first. One example is

> [This professor] has an ability to connect with students that goes beyond anything I have personally experienced. I completed my undergraduate degree at [X university], and in all 4 years I did not have a professor remotely comparable in regard to her commitment to her students and course content. [This professor] goes above and beyond for her students, offering interesting challenges for us to address, and provides priceless professional and personal experience and support. I enjoyed this class more than 95% of the classes I have taken in my career as a student. I am grateful to have had this experience.

This statement assisted me greatly, as it contained aspects of all of my framing questions.

Conclusions

This journey engaged key themes and their counternarratives, which are summarized in Table 11.7. I have learned that nothing replaces the need for

Table 11.7 Summary of Findings: Counternarratives for Pain and Suffering

Key Theme	Social Narrative	Counternarrative	Insights
Visual journals (VJs)	An artistic form of creatively processing thought in the elementary grades.	A reflective agent employing hands, hearts, and minds to think deeply upon ideas.	Being creative is therapeutic, and drawing brings back the child in the reader. It slows down thought.
Stress and anxiety	Society assumes that a mature adult at the university level can master anxiety with previously acquired social skills.	COVID-19 limited or removed hugs, social interaction, and engagement between peers and family.	People cannot flourish in a healthy way without face-to-face social relationships. People need people to thrive.
Pain and suffering	Pain and suffering in a time of normal social engagement is predominantly mediated when family and friends extend love, comfort, support and presence during trials.	Pain and suffering during COVID-19 became an isolated endurance and preoccupation with anxiety when stressors were not mediated, and human distancing was required.	In a pandemic, to combat anxiety professors need to intentionally provide increased engagement and voice between and with students to enable students to feel safe, respected, and heard.
Cultural/social lenses and isms	Modernism, postmodernism, and post-postmodernism engaged human activity and face-to-face conversation.	Transhumanism removes face-to-face interactions and generates human avoidance; replacing being human with technological doing.	Becoming more technologically acute involves becoming less humanly aware and engaged. This damages society interpersonally and economically.
Story and reflection	Engagement with story is therapeutic, distancing the reader from trauma while viewing the plight of another like their own.	In a pandemic, being able to discuss and have voice with others about story is more limited and not as satisfying.	People are living stories and need social engagement to heal and thrive.
The role of education	The knowledge economy informs a person within an area of expertise, to enable a future vocation to be successful.	Education is equipping a person in how to live a life and become a beneficial member of society.	Acquiring wisdom for life requires more than information and skill.

face-to-face social engagement with students, but that intentional planning and the use of VJs for deep reflective, personal engagement and sharing provides a door to hope and healing in a broken and suffering world.

In conclusion, I have personally seen that if students recognize compassion and care in teaching as being an authentic professional stance, then they may be more able to acquire it themselves, saving others from unnecessary pain and suffering in their own classrooms in the future.

References

American Psychological Association. (2021). What's the difference between stress and anxiety? Retrieved from https://www.apa.org/topics/stress/anxiety-difference

Baraister, M. (2014). *Reading and expressive writing with traumatised children, young refugees and asylum seekers: Unpack my heart with words.* Jessica Kingsley Publishers.

Belcher, C., & Loerts, T. (2020). Using visual journals as a reflective worldview window into educator identity. *International Christian Community of Teacher Educators Journal, 15*(1). Retrieved from https://digitalcommons.georgefox.edu/icctej/vol15/iss1/2

Blummer, B. (2015). Some visual literacy initiatives in academic institutions: A literature review from 1999 to the present. *Journal of Visual Literacy, 34*(1), 1–34. https://doi.org/10.1080/23796529.2015.11674721

Boche, B. (2014). Multiliteracies in the classroom: Emerging conceptions of first-year teachers. *Journal of Language and Literacy Education, 10*(1), 114–135. Retrieved from http://jolle.coe.uga.edu

Carlson, R. (2001). Therapeutic use of story in therapy with children. *Guidance and Counseling, 16*, 92–99.

Carr, N. (2010). *The shallows: What the internet is doing to our brains.* W. W. Norton & Company.

Charteris, J. (2014). Epistemological shudders as productive aporia: A heuristic for transformative teacher learning. *International Journal of Qualitative Methods (IJQM), 13*(1), 104–121. https://doi.org/10.1177/160940691401300102

Cornett, C. E., & Cornett, C. F. (1980). *Bibliotherapy: The right book at the right time.* Phi Delta Kappa Educational Foundation.

Forgan, J. (2002). Using bibliotherapy to teach problem solving. *Intervention in School and Clinic, 38*(2), 75–87. https://doi.org/10.1177/10534512020380020201

Gay, C. (2018). *Modern technology and the human future.* InterVarsity Press.

Harris, M. (2014). *The end of absence: Reclaiming what we've lost in a world of constant connection.* HarperCollins Publishing.

Harris, M. (2018, February 9). I have forgotten how to read. *The Globe and Mail.* Retrieved from https://www.theglobeandmail.com/opinion/i-have-forgotten-how-toread/article37921379/?utm_medium=Referrer:+Social+Network+/+Media&utm_campaign=Shared+Web+Article+Links

Jack, S., & Ronan, K. (2008). Bibliotherapy: Practice and research. *School Psychology International*, 161–182. https://doi.org/10.1177/0143034308090058

Korman, G. (2017). *Restart.* Scholastic Press.

Loerts, T., & Belcher, C. (2019). Developing visual literacy competencies while learning course content through visual journaling: Teacher candidate perspectives. *Journal of Visual Literacy*, 38(1–2), 46–65. https://doi.org/10.1080/1051144X.2018.1564603

Lowry, L. (1993). *The giver*. Dell Laurel-Leaf.

Maich, K., Belcher, C., Sider, S., & Johnson, N. (2016). Chapter 36: Using children's literature to support social-emotional growth in the classroom: A bibliotherapeutic approach to education about chronic disease. In Information Resources Management Association (IRMA) *Psychology and mental health: Concepts, methodologies, tools, and applications* (Information Science Reference; 4 Volume Set edition ed., pp. 877–902). IGI Global.

McCulliss, D. (2012). Bibliotherapy: Historical and research perspectives. *Journal of Poetry Therapy*, 25(1), 23–28. https://doi.org/10.1080/08893675.2012.654944

McCulliss, D., & Chamberlain, D. (2013). Bibliotherapy for youth and adolescents— School-based application and research. *Journal of Poetry Therapy*, 26(1), 13–40. https://doi.org/10.1080/08893675.2013.764052

New London Group. (1996). An andragogy of multiliteracies: Designing social futures. *Harvard Educational Review*, 66, 60–92. https://doi.org/10.17763/haer.66.1.17370n67v22j160u

Palmer, P. J. (1998). *The courage to teach: Exploring the Inner landscape of a teacher's life*. Jossey-Bass.

Palmer, P. J. (2000). *Let your life speak*. Jossey-Bass Inc.

Palmer, P. J. (2003). Teaching with heart and soul: Reflections on spirituality in teacher education. *Journal of Teacher Education*, 54(5), 376–476. http://doi.org/10.1177/0022487103257359

Palmer, P. J. (2004). *A hidden wholeness: The journey toward an undivided life*. Jossey-Bass.

Palmer, P. J., & Zajonc, A. (2010). *The heart of higher education: A call to renewal*. Jossey-Bass.

Postman, N. (1988). *Conscientious objections: Stirring up trouble about language, technology and education*. Vintage Books.

Postman, N. (1993). *Technopoly: The surrender of culture to technology*. Vintage Books.

Postman, N. (1995). *The end of education: Redefining the value of school*. Alfred A. Knopf.

Routman, R. (2018). *Literacy essentials: Engagement, excellence and equity for all learners* (2 ed.). Stenhouse Publishers.

Rowsell, J., McLean, C., & Hamilton, M. (2012). Visual literacy as a classroom approach. *Journal of Adolescent and Adult Literacy*, 55(5), 444–447. https://doi.org/10.1002/JAAL.00053

Sachar, L. (1998). *Holes*. Laurel-Leaf books.

Selznick, B. (2008). *The invention of Hugo Cabret*. Scholastic Press.

Smith, D. E. (2005). Chapter 2: Knowing the social: An alternative design. In Dorothy E. Smith.(Ed.), *Institutional ethnography: A sociology for the people* (pp. 27–45). AltaMira Press.

Smith, D. E. (2006). *Institutional ethnography as practice*. Rowman & Littlefield Publishing Group Publishers.

Turkle, S. (2016). *Reclaiming conversation: The power of talk in a digital age.* Penguin Books.

Twenge, J. (2017). *iGen: Why today's super-connected kids are growing up less rebellious, more tolerant, less happy – And completely unprepared for adulthood.* Atria Books.

Walsh, M. (2010). Multimodal literacy: What does it mean for classroom practice? *Australian Journal of Language and Literacy, 33,* 211–239.

Wright, N. T. (1996). *The original Jesus: The life and vision of a revolutionary.* Eerdmans's Publishing Company.

Zusak, M. (2005). The book thief. Alfred A. Knopf.

Appendix A

BOX 11.1 STUDENT INSTRUCTIONS ON VJS

To reduce stress on repeatedly reading the syllabus, in the week prior to your Monday night class I engaged a visual journal (VJ) (Blummer, 2015; New London Group, 1996; Roswell et al., 2012; Walsh, 2010).

Example of a Weekly Visual Journal

Your task is in the green box for class tonight

GOALS:
1. Exploring the genre of the graphic novel
2. Identify how reading and viewing differ
3. Submit your VJ pre-assignment to be used in class lit circles and be ready to discuss it
4. How did the story make you feel and why?

Reflections: 2 students (one prior and one after mid class)

Book Talks: 3 students (5 min. each)

How does the postmodern graphic novel usher in and relate to life now?

Genre: Graphic Novel

Class Outline: QUESTION of the DAY greetng!

- *Reflective thoughts: Student*
- *Book Talk #1 - Student*
- *Share pre-assignments feedback from reading by Harris and the structure of a graphic postmodern novel.*
- *Lit circle on Hugo Cabret and movie comparison (share reflective VJs / Harris Article in literature circles)*
- *Book Talk #2 – Student*
  BREAK
- *Reflective thoughts: Student*
- *Book Talk #3 - Student*
- *Postmodern lit as a worldview paradigm and literary device (PPT sent in advance)*
- *Graphic literature as an expression of a philosophical condition regarding the act of reading: discussion*
- *Next class Nov. 3: read/respond to the book The Giver*
- *Reflective thoughts: Nov. 3 = name of student*

1. Read Hugo Cabret and submit 1 pre-class VJ assignment by email before Monday night
2. Book talks

To think about:

How do you experience the views of Harris?
- Bring your VJ to show similarity and difference between book and movie, and your preference.
- How does reading format affect the mind?

Harris, M. (2018, February 9), I Have Forgotten How to Read. *The Globe and Mail.* **Submit by email.**

https://www.theglobeandmail.com/opinion/i-have-forgotten-how-toread/article37921379/

Belcherism: Philosophical reflection: If we are to be human 'beings', not just humans 'doing', how do we not become merely a mirror of what our culture values at any given time? Do we become automata?

Figure 11.1 Example of a weekly visual journal.

A visual journal (VJ) is a form of graphic organizer containing a balance of visuals and print to engage students in a clear and condensed format. This one-page document provides you, my student, with requirements for the next class. For instructive purposes, I implemented a design of VJ that instructs, provokes voice and thought, and engages intentional participation. Our learning community will engage VJs in this class in two forms.

The VJ will be a weekly instructional device and will also be used creatively as a reflective mirror for learning and thought you have reflected upon from assigned readings. VJs are similar to graphic organizers, word webs, and charts – except they contain one major difference. As author of a VJ assignment, you will represent learning pictorially, and then reflectively state in written form what thinking led you to choose the images within your individual work. An example of a VJ is included in Appendix A, Figure 11.1.

12 Poetic Justice

Healing and Disrupting Systemic Oppression in Education through Critical Pedagogy

Ardavan Eizadirad

We hope you have enjoyed engaging with the various topics and methodologies covered in this book, and that you took some time to pause and reflect on your own pain and suffering, particularly when, where, and how you would share your pain and suffering with others in an authentic way that can be therapeutic and transformative. These are conversations that need ongoing discussions. Therefore, we hope as a reader through your journey of engaging with this book and its ideas, you feel part of the community that with intentionality and resiliency will disrupt oppression in educational contexts and advocate for counternarratives of pain and suffering as critical pedagogy. We conclude this book with a poem written by Ardavan Eizadirad bringing together the big ideas and themes discussed:

The language of pain and suffering is universal,
a starting point for empathy and understanding.
Recognizing that you are not alone, and beginning the journey to heal,
and be an agent of social change.

But the system wants to keep you down,
and tell you "Don't be emotional,"
"Be professional,"
"This is not the place for the emotions to be expressed." Or is it?
Who decides?
What should you share?
With whom?
When and where?
In what ways?
What will be the consequences?
Who does your silence benefit?

Forgetting for now might be the best tactic for survival,
because at times living and doing equity work can be exhausting.
It drains your emotions.

DOI: 10.4324/9781003205296-15

But in communities that foster brave spaces, we experience belonging.
This facilitates remembering with a purpose.
We can begin to be even more courageous in the face of our fears and
anxieties.
We shall overcome, but at our own pace.
We shall speak up, but on our own terms.
Keeping it real and staying authentic to who we are and our values.
If we choose to do so, we shall share our pain and suffering,
and our past and on-going traumas and microaggressions experienced,
to disrupt with intentionality.
To question the norm and who it privileges.
Who does it silence and mute? For what reasons?
Who does it hyper-visibilize and whose existence, opinions,
perspectives, and lived experiences does it dismiss?

As much as it's a personal journey,
let's not forget the root causes of such oppressions.
SYSTEMIC oppression and inequities.
Pain and suffering, perpetuated by inequality of access to
opportunities.

Let us share our pain and suffering as critical pedagogy,
so we can heal and hope for change.
and disrupt oppression in education.

Forgive, for yourself first and foremost. Then forgive for others.
Support one another and work in solidarity,
to call out injustice, oppression, unfairness, and exploitation.
Create networks and coalitions and to collectively fight unjust systems,
and their policies, practices, programs, and processes which
systemically disadvantage marginalized identities, families, and
communities.

In community, we can heal, hope, and do transformative work.
Find brave spaces to share our authentic selves,
including our pain and suffering.
This is part of your journey: who you are, and who you are becoming.
Embrace your emotions and feelings,
good and bad.
Sometimes we learn more from losing than winning.
Sometimes we learn more from the pain and the joy.

Learn from trauma.
Learn from your own trauma

Learn from others' trauma.
Deconstruct it layer by layer,
What is it trying to tell you?

Listen,
Learn,
Unlearn,
Relearn.
Revisit the pain and suffering.
What is it trying to tell you now from a new perspective?

The struggle guides us in new directions.
Identify the why behind your practices and how you present yourself
to others.
Why do it this way? Is there an alternative way that might be better?
What message does it send?

Embrace and indulge in the pain and suffering.
Harness energy and purpose from it,
but of course, when you are ready, at your own pace.

Decolonize your imagination,
your ideas,
heart, mind, and soul.
Be an ally where you can.
As educators and community activists, decolonize research and
publication policies and practices.
Question the norm so it becomes abnormal.
Disrupt with intentionality and through storytelling,
so that we can decolonize the system.

Use critical pedagogy as a tool,
to center community,
solidarity,
activism,
advocacy,
coalition-building, and
grassroot community needs and voices.

Create time to love yourself.
Self-care.
Love yourself and your community.
Strategize.
Mobilize.

Find spiritual nourishment in your passions and interests, and thrive in caring and supportive relationships.

Give gratitude.
Respect different opinions and lived experiences.
Do not judge, but seek to understand,
including the complexities and nuances it involves.
Make the conversation about the system and not the individual.

Celebrate small successes.
Overcome barriers.
Rest.
Take a deep breath.

Forget,
remember,
share.

Share,
remember,
forget.

Remember the pain, anger, and frustrations.
Remember the joy, happiness, and laughter.
Truth-telling can be empowering and transformative.
Tell your truth,
in your own words and style,
at your own pace.
Call it out.
SCREAM,
whisper,
SHOUT,
sit and reflect in silence.
There is no right way.
Do it the way it works for you,
to heal and hope.

Invest in your spiritual growth.
Imagine the impossible. How can you make it possible?
Share your sacrifices.
Set goals.
Create an action plan.
Work hard.
Go get it!

Revisit goals. Revaluate if needed.
Accomplish.
Repeat.

Create time for rest and rejuvenation.
Find a mentor and caring support networks,
in person or online remotely.

Tell your story without censorship with the pain and suffering
included.
#KeepItReal
#RealRecognizeReal
Amplify your voice and your experiences with intentionality.

Hope is contagious.
Sharing pain and suffering as critical pedagogy generates hope,
and disrupts systemin oppression in education with a purpose.
You are not alone.

We are not alone.
Together, we can prosper and change the system to center equity and
social justice,
not as a counter-narrative,
but as THE narrative.

With love, respect, and gratitude,
we shall overcome.

Index

Page numbers in **bold** represent tables, while page numbers in *italics* represent figures, photographs or images.

able/disabled binaries 53
ableism, and social justice spaces 61
Aboud, Gary 109
Absolon, K. 96–97
academic aunties 83–84, 87n6
academic institutions, acknowledging interconnectedness 84
academic spaces: assumed narratives in 25; racism in 105; silencing in 72–75, 82, 114; women in 76
academic work, as "worth" 6
activism/advocacy: adverse consequences of 115; in assignments 30–31
activism stances 24
Adams, John 40
Adichie, Chimamanda Ngozi 46
African American feminist thought 106–107
African Canadian experiences, *vs.* African American 107
African Canadian feminist theories 106–107
African Diaspora 40, 108
Alberta: Aboriginal Studies 30 164, 166, 168–171, 176; educational policies 152–153; "Growing Faculty, Staff and Student Foundational Knowledge of Indigenous Philosophies, Epistemologies, Ontologies, and Pedagogies" 145–146, 159; *Leadership Quality Standard* 144; *Teaching Quality Standard* 144
All about Love: New Visions (hooks) 67

allies 144
American Psychological Association 182
America's Lie 40–41
Anderson, E. 99
Anderson, K. 73–74
andragogy 183, 192
Andrew **129**, 130
anger 2, 32–33
anthropocentric curricula 164–165
anti-racism 21, 117; in education 127; and healing 164
anxiety 182, 184, 188
Arao, B. 24, 30
Arbery, Ahmaud 48
Armstrong, J. 73–74
artworks *75, 81, 85; see also* poetry
Ashmun Institute 41
Ashraf al-Makhluqat 166–167, 175
assessment, attitudes towards 31
assimilation, expectations of 111
Atcheynum, Chauntelle 169, 172, 176–177
Auger, Charis 143–161
authenticity: and storytelling 16; teachers 185
authentic selves, as counternarratives 6, 7–8, 9–12
autobiographical writing 22
autoethnography 107; Black feminist 107

baby elephant syndrome 28–30
Baraister, M. 185
Basso, K. H. 77
Batin 167

Battiste, M. 155
Beagan, B. L. 105
Belcher, Christina 182–194
Bell, Derrick 42
belonging, encouraging 26–28
bibliotherapy 185
Bissell, A. 97–98
Black colleges/universities 41, 123
Black communities 39; destruction of 39; oppression of 39; Tulsa riots 38–39
Black cultures, presumed homogeneity of 111–112
Black educators 130–132, 135
Black feminist thought 106–107
Black history: in Canada 112–114; erased 111–114, 116, 123
Black History Month 105, 127
Black Lives Matter movement (BLM) 45
Blackness, understanding 112–113
Black students 116; and activism 114–115; discrimination against 122; groups for 130–131; marginalization of 124–125; at primarily White institutions 105; racial profiling of 125–126, 130–133; supporting 114–116, 131–132
Black Wall Street 38, 46–47
Blimkie, M. 98
Bonila-Silva, E. 127
The Book Thief (Zusak) 191, **192**
Bourdain, Anthony 109
Bourdieu, P. 20
Brand, Dionne 64, 108, 110, 117–118
brave spaces 19–21, 23, 27, 34; and baby elephant syndrome 29–30; creating 32; guidelines for 25–26; and risk-taking 24–25, 27, 32; as safe spaces 27
Breault, R. A. 22
Brockwood, Evelyn 158
Brown, A. 116
Brown, L. 159
Brown vs. Board of Education 42–43
bullies/bullying 76–77
bundles 174
Butler-Kisber, L. 75

Calderon, D. 98
call to action 33
Campbell, Andrew B. 1–12, 19–35
Canada: Bill C-31 149, 160n3; Black history in 112–114; COVID-19 in 91–92; education system in 125; higher education in 52, 110–111, 117, 144–145; Indian Act of 1876 100; Indigenous silencing in 72–75; international students 115, 117; and the Klu Klux Klan 113; presumed homogeneity of Black cultures 111–112; racial profiling in 125–126; racism in 105–107, 111; and slavery 113, 124; and teacher education 101; Truth and Reconciliation Commission (TRC) 144, 149, 170–171; White Paper of 1969 100; *see also* Alberta; New Brunswick; Nova Scotia; Ontario; Prince Edward Island
Canadian residential schools 102, 143; unmarked graves at 2, 144
capitalism, and IESL 55–56, 60–61
Cardinal, Bob 166
Carr-Stewart, S. 100
Carter, L. M. 76
Casey 58–59
cellphilm 114
ceremonial Circles 147, 156; Medicine Circle 148
ceremonies, and learning 155
Chamberlain, D. 185
Charis 148–150
Charteris, J. 186
Chauvin, Derek 2, 41
Civil Rights Era 43, 45
Civil Rights Movement, and "We Shall Overcome" 40
classrooms: Ardavan on 26–27; building inclusive 44; decolonization of 20
Clemens, K. 24, 30
Codjoe, H. M. 126
collages 74, *75*
collective resistance, and social media 68
Collins, Patricia Hill 106
colonization/colonialism 100–101; in education 110; impacts of 149–150; perpetuated in universities 152; in Trinidad and Tobago 108–109
Colour of Poverty–Colour of Change 126
comfort zones, growing beyond 26
communities of care 84
concussions 188
confidence 185
connection, and vulnerability 5

Conscientious Objections
(Postman) 190
consciousness 164–165
Cook-Sather, A. 24, 32
Cooper, Anna Julia 41
coping mechanisms: forgetting 20;
silence 20
counternarratives **193**; authentic selves
as 6, 7–8 , 9–12; Belcher's course as
184; brave spaces as 34; centering 4,
22–23; in CRT 43, 45; encouraging
15; lived experiences as 21–22;
poetry as 72; preparing educators
for 43–46; self-location as 96–99;
and social media 68; telling/reliving
trauma as 69; Tulsa Race Massacre
47; *see also* self-location
COVID-19 64, 182, 190; educational
impacts 93–94; and restructuring
education 91
creation 34
Cree language 71, 80, 87, 165, 169
Crenshaw, Kimberlé 42
critical literacy 183
critical pedagogy 128; and disabling
narratives 63; and IESL programs 54;
of lived experiences 87; pain/suffering
as 1, 3, 21–23
critical race theory (CRT) 19, 22, 126–
127; and duoethnology 23; overview
41–43; politicization of 42–43, 48
Cudjoe, S. R. 109
cultural/language loss 151
cultural lenses **190**
culturally relevant instruction 44
culturally responsive pedagogy 43,
174–175
curriculum development, minority
representation in 127

Danaher, P. A. 116
David **129**, 130–131
Davis, D. 75
decolonization: of classrooms/education
20, 84, 96, 99; of self-location 95,
98; of settler thinking 92–93, 95–96
deficit thinking 34, 131
Dei, G. 125, 129–130
Delgado, R. 126–127
Dénommé-Welch, S. 100–101
Derek Chauvin trial 2
Desai, M. 101
DiAngelo, Robin 134
Diaspora journal 1

disability, social model of 57
disabling narratives 53, 56, 63
disruption from within 34
Dobbin, F. 134
Donald, Dwayne 140, 170–171, 176
Drawson, A. 95
DuBois, W.E.B. 41
duoethnography 19, 22
duoethnology, and critical race theory
(CRT) 23
dystopian novels **191**

education: "banking concept" 128;
Canadian system 125; colonialism
in 110; and connection 177–178;
decolonization of 20, 84, 96, 99,
144–145; Eurocentric focus of 123,
127; Freire on 112; gifted students
126; inequities in 92; and Jim Crow
41; and liberal philosophy 163, 165;
mainstream 102; neoliberal models of
6, 21, 23, 25, 27, 175; politicization
of 42–44, 48; power dynamics in 26,
29, 52; racism in 49; restructuring of
91; and self-location 99–100, 102;
settler/colonial biases in 84; and
silencing 72–75
educators: in Canada 101; and
COVID-19 91–92; diversity gap 135;
lack of Black educators 130, 135;
responsibilities of 46; role of 91, 128
Eizadirad, Ardavan 1–12, 19–35,
199–203; tattoos 7–8
Ellis, eginald K. 38–50
embodied experiences 71–72
emotional sharing 67–68; institutional
regulation of 6, 15, 23; personal
control over 33
emotions: embracing 67; as weakness 21
Encyclopedia of the Qur'an 167
End of Education (Postman) 190
Ennser-Kananen, J. 4
Equal Employment Opportunities
Commission (EEOC) lawsuits 42
equity, talking about 28
Ermine, Willie 155, 157
ethical discourse 114–115;
dissemination of 116
ethical spaces 157–158
ethnography 186

Faces from the Bottom of the Well
(Bell) 42
Fain, K. 38

Faulkner, S. L. 71–72
Favors, Jelani 41
feminism, changing understanding of 59–60
feminist theory 106
"Filipina/o American" experience 101
Floyd, George 48
forgetting pedagogy 3
Foucault, M. 55
Franklin, Benjamin 40
Franklin, Buck Colbert 38–39
Franklin, John Hope 38, 41
Franklin, Mollie Parker 38
Freire, P. 30, 109, 112, 116, 128

Gadamer, H.-G. 172
gatekeepers 15; institutional regulations as 15–16, 23
Gaudry, A. 144–145
Gay, Geneva 44–45
gifted students 126
Gilmour, G. I. 20, 24, 31–32
The Giver (Lowry) 191
global citizenship 53, 55
Global South, learning about 52
Gonzalez, I. 98–99
good relations 71
guidance counsellors 132–133

Halagao, P. E. 101
Hanna, K. B. 21, 25, 30
Hanohano, Peter 167–168
healing 177; and anti-racism 164; and self-location 99; and silence 67; and tears 158
Henry, F. 105
Henry, Frances 110
Herrmann, J. 24
hierarchical power relations 4
Hill, Lauryn 33
Holes (Sachar) 188
holism 164–165, 170, 176, 178; and self-location 98
hooks, bell 2, 67, 76, 106, 115
Hunter 60–61

Iaquinta, T. 4
"I Get Out" (Hill) 33
Indigenous communities 151; and oral traditions 102; raised profile of 144; and spirituality 93
Indigenous education: decolonization of 99; and the Indian Act (1876) 100; learning processes 155; White Paper of 1969 100

Indigenous history: erased 123, 143; lack of knowledge of 100–101; misrepresentation of 97, 101; silencing 72–75
"An Indigenous Pedagogy for Colonization" (Wisselink) 103
Indigenous research 153–154, 156; lack of accomodation for 153, 159; scrutiny of 152–153; and self-location 96–97; *vs.* Western paradigms 153–154
Indigenous Story Method 148, 156–157
Indigenous students 143
Indigenous ways of knowing 143; self-education about 84
inner dwelling 177
intentional silences 26
interconnectedness 173; need to acknowledge 84
Intercordia program 53–56; mentorship in 61–63; research into 56–57; and vulnerability 53–54, 57–63
intergenerational narrative reverberations 149
intergenerational trauma 48, 100, 102, 149
international experiential service learning (IESL): and Canada 52; Intercordia program 53–56; narratives about 52, 55–56, 60; Northern subjects in 53, 57–58, 60, 63; organizations 52; research into 56–57; student narratives from 54; and vulnerability 53–54, 57–63
international students 110; Black 107, 111, 114–115; growing numbers of 117
The Invention of Hugo Cabret (Selznick) **189**
The Invisible Student in the Jamaican Classroom, Campbell 9–10
Islam 168, 170, 178; *see also* Rumi
Islamophobia 164
isolation 58–59; and Blackness 110

James, Alissa 169, 172, 176
Jamie 59–60
Janes, D. P. 76
Jefferess, David 53
Jefferson, Thomas 40
Jim Crow 39; and education 41; and Trinidad and Tobago 108
Jiwa, Shainool 175
Jones, A. H. 117

Jones, Ralph 40
journaling *see* visual journals
June, Lyla 67
Justin 110

Kana 61–62
Karakose, T. 92
Kasamali, Zahra 163–178
Kelley, R. D. G. 115
Kendi, I. X. 43
Kim, Y. K. 117
Kincey, Sundra D. 38–50; personal
   experiences of 49
King, Martin Luther Jr. 41
knowledge: destabilizing 63; Indigenous
   102, 143–144, 151, 154–156, 160
Korteweg, L. 97–98
Kouri, S. 92–93
Kovach, M. 92, 95–96
Kulnieks, A. 155

Ladson-Billings, Gloria 45
Lafferty, Anita 71–87
Lake Couchiching 151
Lambe, J. 102
land-based education 98
language, and memory 139–140
Laprise, M. 143
learning, and ceremonies 155
Legette, K. B. 130
Leonardo, Z. 23
lived experiences: of marginalization
   143; recognizing 86–87
Lopez, R. G. 22
Lorde, Audre 2–3, 72
Lorenz, D. 144–145
Lorenz, D. E. 118
*Love and Compassion: Exploring Their
   Role in Education* (Miller) 5
Lumsden, Daniel 122–136
Lyle, E. 22

McAuliffe, J. D. 167
McCulliss, D. 185
McGaa, E. 167–168
Madison, D. 24
Madison, James 40
"Mamwlad" (June) 67
Mandela, Nelson 50
Maracle, L. 73–74
Marandola, Kateri Marie 91–103
Marshall, Thurgood 41–42
matriarchs 73–75, 80, 81, 87; learning
   from 77–78

Matthews, Levi 169, 172, 176–177
Maynard, Robyn 125–126
mental health 130
mentorship: and Black students 105,
   111; importance of 82; loss of 105;
   and Trinidad and Tobago 108;
   University of Alberta 151–152; and
   vulnerability 62–64
métissage 169–171
Michael **129**, 132
microaggressions 133–134; from
   teachers 28; *see also* systemic racism
Miller, J. P. 5
Mogadime, D. 111
Mohamed, T. 105
Montero, M. K. 100–101
Mooney, Julie A. 71–87
movies, *vs.* novels **189**
Murray, Pauli 42
Murrell, P. 128
Mwangi, George 116

narratives of oppression, muting 4
narrators, awareness of 4
National Association for the
   Advancement of Colored People
   (NAACP) 42
Native Americans 43
neoliberalism: in education 6, 21,
   23, 25, 27, 175; in IESL programs
   60–61; resisting 63
New Brunswick: and the Klu Klux Klan
   113; notable Black people from 113;
   slavery in 124
9/11 attacks 163–164
non-verbal communication 77
Noreiga, Alicia 105–118; background
   107–108
Nova Scotia, slavery in 124
novels, *vs.* movies **189**

objective reality 23
objectivity 97
online literacy course: assignments
   183–184; questions for 184–186,
   187; shared activities 186; syllabus
   alterations 183
Ontario 125; Black students in 122,
   125–126, 132; education systems
   in 125–126; Equity and Inclusive
   Education Strategy 122, 134;
   teacher diversity in 135; Toronto
   District School Board (TDSB) 126,
   132–133

Ontario Centre of Excellence for Child and Youth Mental Health 174
oportunities, inequality of 25
oppression: of Black communities 39; seen as "past" 127; and trauma 149
#OppressionOlympics 5
oppressive practices, challenging 5
oral traditions 68, 80–81; Indigenous 102, 155; *see also* storytelling
O'Ree, Willie 113
Osman, A. A. 128
overcoming silence 3

pain: intergenerational nature of 48; masking/avoiding 140; processing 139
Paine, R. 163
Palmer, Parker 185
panel discussions: facilitating 114–116; issues with 116
participation, Ardavan on 26–27
participatory research 156; cellphilm 114; lack of accommodation for 153
Parts Unknown 109
Payne, Charles M. 49
pedagogies of pain/suffering, increased interest in 1–2
Pedagogy of the Oppressed (Freire) 128
Peltier, Sharla Mskokii 143–161
Peltier, Stan 146, 150, 152
Place to Belong (Mooney) 84, *85*, 86
poetic rhythms 71
poetry 72–74, 76–78, 80–81, 83–87, 172–173, 175–176, 199–203; and self-location 94; *see also* artworks
post-secondary education, and Black educators 130
prairies *79*
Prince Edward Island, slavery in 124
publishing 32

Quebec, students in 125–126
questions: to ask students **187**; on anxiety 184–185; on confidence 186; "Growing Faculty, Staff and Student Foundational Knowledge of Indigenous Philosophies, Epistemologies, Ontologies, and Pedagogies" 145; on war 191, **192**; and self-location 95
Qur'anic teachings 166

race, conversations about 44
racialized identities: institutional gatekeeping of 23; and required sharing 28–29

racialized subjectivity 23
racism 127; in academic spaces 105; in Canada 105–107, 111; in education 49; and Trinidad and Tobago 108–109; *see also* systemic racism
rahma 175
Razack, N. 57
relational models, in IESL 54–56
relationship building, and storytelling 16
reserves 154; living conditions on 102
Restart (Korman) 188
Reynolds, G. 113
Richardson, Arthur St. George 113
risk-taking: and brave spaces 24–25, 27, 32; teachers modelling 21–22
Routman, Reggie 185
Rugat, E. J. 128
Rumi 67, 165, 171–176

Sabga-Aboud, Mario 109
sacred ecology 164–168, 176
safe spaces 19, 21, 25, 34, 115; Andrew on 27; brave spaces as 27; need for 20; and open discussions 47
Salvador, Rose 169, 172, 174–175, 177
Sameshima, P. 71
segregation 48; in New Brunswick 113
self-healing 15; and storytelling 15–16; variable times for 20
self-knowledge 103
self-location 92–94, 102–103; as counternarrative 96–99; and decolonization 95, 98; and education 99–100, 102; and healing 99; and Indigenous research 96–97; and questions 95; and trauma 99–100
self-loss 177
self-management 99
settler thinking: decolonizing 92–93, 95–96; in education 84
Seven Fallen Feathers: Racism, Death, and Hard Truths in a Northern City (Talaga) 101–102
sexism 76
Shadow of Myself, No More (Mooney) 82, 83
Shakir, Ameenah 38–50
shame 150
Sider, Steve 1–12, 139–141
silence: imagery of 74–75; intentional 26; overcoming 68–69; reasons for 67; writings about 72
silencing: in education 72–75, 82; recovering from 78
Simpson, L. B. 73–74

slavery 40; in Canada 124; and Canadian history 113; narratives about 124
Smith, D. 186
social justice conversations 21; in education 127
social justice spaces, and ableism 61
social lenses **190**
social media 68
Solitary: Unbroken by Four Decades in Solitary Confinement. My Story of Transformation and Hope (Woodfox) 5
South, *othering* 55–58
spokesperson identities, and racialized identities 29
Spray, W. A. 113
Stefancic, J. 126–127
Stonehouse, Jodi 174
storytelling 2; and authenticity 16; autobiographical writing 22; and Black Americans 46; and brave spaces 20; and calls to action 33; cultural preservation through 15–16; invoking 15; listener expectations for 26; and relationship building 16; and self-healing 15; by Talaga 101–102; of triumph 46; *see also* oral traditions
Strega, S. 159
stress 192; coping with 188
stress triggers 184
structural racism 41; *see also* critical race theory (CRT)
struggles, normality of 61–62
students, exploitation of 32
subjective experiences of reality 23
Subranmanian, S. 91–92
systemic oppression: Alberta universities 146; and lack of support from teachers 28; and telling/reliving trauma 24; understanding 31–32
systemic racism: Canadian education systems 125; and Canadian universities 110–111; dismantling 134–135; *see also* racism

Talaga, Tanya 101–102
Tator, C. 105
Taylor, Breonna 40–41, 48
Teaching Lodges 146, *147*, 148, 150, 152, 154, 156–157, *158*, 160
Teaching to Transgress (hooks) 115
Technopoly (Postman) 190
telling/reliving trauma 3; as counternarrative 69; expectations around 26; harm through 16–17,

29–30; and institutional gatekeeping 16; lived experiences 21; and systemic oppression 24
Tindley, Charles Albert 40
To Kill a Mockingbird (Lee) 123–124
transhumanism 190
traumatic experiences: and forgetting 139–140; of oppression 149; revisiting 68; and self-location 99–100
Trinidad and Tobago 107–110, 112
trust 4–5; and brave spaces 24
Tulsa 48
Tulsa Race Massacre 38–39, 46–47
Turner, D. A. 163
Turner, T. 135

Underground Railroad 113, 124
University of Alberta Elder Protocol document 151–153
un-silencing 71

Venn, C. 163
Verduzco-Baker, L. 29
visual journals 182, 185–186, 188, 191, **193**, 194, *197*, 198
Vizina, Yvonne 157
Vorstermans, Jessica 52–64
Vrasti, W. 55, 60–61
vulnerability: Campbell and Eizadirad on 23; and connection 5; and IESL programs 53–54, 57–63; and mentorship 62–64; narratives about 59; transformative nature of 33–34

Walker, Abraham Beverley 113
Walker, J. W. G. 113
Wane, N. N. 106
water 173
Watson, Allyson L. 38–50; personal experiences 48
Wayskapeeyos/Oshkaabewisag 151–152, 160n4
Weiner, E. 30
"We Shall Overcome" 40
Western academic institutions 76
Western research paradigms, *vs.* Indigenous 153–154
White Fragility (DiAngelo) 134
Whiteness: and beauty standards 29; as ideology 21; as norm 118
white supremacy, in education 127
Whitfield, H. A. 124
wicihitowin 71, 87
Willett, C. 96–97

Winslow, Mary Matilda 113
Wisselink, K. 103
women: in academia 76; in CRT 42;
    silencing by 76; silencing of 80
women's history, silencing 72–75
Woodfox, Albert 5, 68
Woodson, Carter G. 41
Wright, N. T. 184

written assignments 30; and self-
    location 94

Young 149
Young, Darius J. 38–50

Zahir 167
Zimmerman, George 41

Milton Keynes UK
Ingram Content Group UK Ltd.
UKHW050146260424
441726UK00014B/90

9 781032 070889